Positive Flow Childbirth

by
Lawrence Vijay Girard

FruitgardenPublishing

"Information and Inspiration
for Living in Harmony with Life."

First Printing 2012

Front cover baby photo by
Louise Ivy

Back cover baby photo
the day after the birth of
Kai and Sabari.

ISBN-10: 098489621X
ISBN-13: 9780984896219

DEDICATED

to Bhavani for the gift of her friendship
to Sabari and Kai who arrived and live with style
to Swami Kriyananda my friend and guide

Authors Note

This book was originally published in 1995 as *Doorway to a New Lifetime: Childbirth from a Spiritual View*. I still feel this is a part of life to which people don't give sufficient spiritual attention. In this new edition I have made surprisingly few changes given the time that has lapsed. The reason is that spiritual principles don't change over time, it is our application of those principles to the unique circumstances of our lives that is ever new. Never-the-less, I hope that a new title and some sprucing up will reenergize interest in this sacred subject.

Dear Reader

This book is intended as a spiritual guide - not as a medical guide - for understanding the various issues surrounding childbirth. Discussion of medical issues and how to approach them from a spiritual point of view should not be construed as medical advice. For answers to medical questions you should consult a medical professional.

Contents

Preface

It was on a cool winter evening in the 1970's that I found myself outside looking in through the living room window of a small wooden cabin in the foothills of the Sierra Nevada. I was kneeling on a foam pad with my face as close to the window as I could get it - without steaming up the view. I was transfixed by the events that were taking place within the small room.

My good friend Alan was sitting by his wife, Heath, who had a look of deep concentration on her face. She was drawing on energies deep within herself and Alan was encouraging her. Heath had been in labor for over 12 hours and she was tired. Penny, the midwife, was monitoring her vital signs. Although things were going a bit slowly, everything was still within the parameters that Penny considered safe. In my mind I reviewed the circumstances that had brought me to this unexpected perch.

Alan and Heath had invited me to attend the birth of their child. But when I arrived at their small cabin it was so crowded with items for the birth there really hadn't been room for me. We decided that when the time came I would watch from outside. Even though Alan had assured me that I was welcome, it did seem a little strange to be looking in through the living room window. But when Alan smiled at me as I watched, I felt reassured.

The evening sky was clear and the forest quiet. The air was pungent with the smell of cedar and pine from the surrounding forest, which mingled with the rising smoke from the wood stove. While time passed I thought how different this was from the image of birth that I had been brought up with.

As a child, the only exposure to childbirth that I can remember is from television. You know, a woman lying on a hospital gurney as she is hurriedly raced down a brightly lit corridor while she screams her head off and then disappears through the sacred double doors that only hospital staff can use. The husband is ushered into a waiting room, where he alternately sits with clenched jaw or paces back and forth across the small smoke filled room.

Then, it is back to the delivery room where you can see contortions of pain on the mothers face. With a final yell that no doubt strikes fear in the hearts of many mothers to be, the happy moment comes. The doctor smiles knowledgeably and pronounces the gender of the child. The mother then falls into an exhausted slumber as the baby is taken away to some unseen place. The father, having been notified, fulfills his part of the birthing ritual by grinning, while handing out cigars to anyone who happens to be in the area.

Now, for the first time in my just over 20 years of life, I was watching an actual birth. There was nothing impersonal or antiseptic about it. Both father and mother were doing their allotted parts to manage the needs of the moment and there was an aura of harmony and peacefulness that radiated from the unfolding drama. Heath was now pushing for all she was worth. Even though she was exhausted you could tell from her expression that she was determined and in control of herself. I found myself entering into her efforts and mentally offering her what strength I could.

As the birth became imminent Alan moved from Heaths' side into position so that he could be the one to welcome the child into this world with his own hands. When the head appeared Alan's eyes grew wide with wonder. He reached to support the little head with his hands as it began to emerge. Alan's face beamed with excitement. Once the head was out it was only a few more moments. There was one final push from Heath: then there was a little baby boy being lovingly held by his father.

The midwife reached over with a suction device to clear the baby's mouth of fluid. As soon as the mouth became clear we could all see the first breath of air entering into the little body, animating it with the breath of independent physical life.

With that first breath I was filled with a thrill that I shall never forget. A new life had emerged into this world. It was as elemental as the making of the creation itself. I felt in some subtle way connected to all of the souls that had come before this little baby, along with those still yet to come; eternally joined in the sacred lineage that we call humankind. I was awestruck at the thought of the universal forces that can bring such an incredible thing to pass. It must be a closed mind and heart, indeed, which can be present at the birth of a child and not perceive the miracle of it.

After cutting and tying the umbilical cord with Penny's help, Alan wrapped his son in a soft blanket and placed him on Heath's chest. Mother and father then enveloped their little boy in the powerfully radiating warmth of their overflowing love.

As I left them to their joy I was aware of the honor it had been to have shared this very special moment with my good friends. It was only after actually seeing the struggle, witnessing the victory of that first breath, and feeling the sacred vibration that filled the room, that I began to become aware of a small portion of the power and glory of human birth.

Since that very special day so long ago I have often wondered why so little attention is given to the spiritual side of such a momentous event. While much focus has been given by our society to the physical aspects of birth, the opportunities for greater spiritual understanding that can be gained from a close look at childbirth are not often enough explored.

Even though one of the most important keys to success in the spiritual life is to include God in every moment of every experience, it happens all too often that we put our spiritual life on hold while we deal with intense life experiences. Then we resume our spiritual efforts when we "have the time". Remember, it is only through constant inner association with the Divine that we can begin to really explore our spiritual realities.

If we want to achieve our highest spiritual potential, we need to be ever vigilant in our efforts to integrate the time that we give to the demands and challenges of this world, with the time that we allow ourselves for achieving our spiritual goals.

Today, the advances of technology have taken much of the mystery out of childbirth. If you want, you can find out the sex of your baby before it is even born. With induced labors and Cesarean Sections you can virtually choose the day and time of the birth. Certainly it is more common today than ever before for individuals to make more of the choices about birthing issues, still, it is all too common for expectant parents to hand over decision making to the doctor. And of course, doctors are usually involved only after the most important decision of all has been made; which is, whether or not have a child in the first place!

The idea of consciously making decisions in our lives is an essential component of approaching life spiritually. While Gods' existence is not dependent upon our opinion, our ability to perceive God's presence and His will for us, is very much up to us. While it is true that God never imposes upon the freedom of the soul to ignore truth, remember, the door to spiritual understanding is always open to those who are interested. All we need to do is activate our desire to know truth by consciously and actively seeking it. It is in the act of trying to attune ourselves to Spirit that we open up the lines of communication with our higher spiritual nature.

Contrary to the beliefs of many, living the spiritual life is not based on the passive following of proscribed rules. It is based on experience: personal and direct. While on our spiritual quest we often receive valuable guidance and inspiration from teachers and sacred writings. At the same time, we must be careful to distinguish between our own personal perception of life and God, and the living of life based strictly on the opinions of others.

It isn't enough to say that something is true because the scriptures, my teacher or any other source says it is so; we need to realize truth directly for ourselves. Otherwise, we may be led astray by well-meaning people who simply do not know that they don't know - thus, the classic case of the blind leading the blind. And even more importantly, we may mistake the amassing of intellectual knowledge for true self-realization.

There is much in this world that would have us believe that it is in the fulfilling of all of our desires that we will find happiness. Society tries to convince us of this through every advertisement. But where is the real joy and fulfillment that this world offers? Those who have reached the pinnacle of any endeavor know how fleeting their joy can be.

Positive Flow Childbirth

The soul longs for a permanent solution to all suffering and to experience unending happiness. Where can this be found? There is only one place. The custodians of the highest truths – the saints of all religions – have proclaimed that the direct personal experience of God is the solution to all life challenges and the fulfillment of all desires.

It will be my purpose in this book to explore with you the connection between the underlying principles of the spiritual life and the many issues associated with childbirth. What I am offering is a framework, based on the principles of the spiritual life, from which you can make your decisions pertaining to the birth experience.

It is my sincere hope that as you read this book, you will get not only practical information that can help you in your life, but that you will also capture a glimmer of the soul-thrilling energy that is present at the birth of a child. For the coming into this world of a soul is a doorway to the most profound of all subjects: life itself.

Chapter 1

The Mystery of Life

For many, procreation is a primal urge that is second only to the instinct for survival itself. To these people, the natural continuation of the species, Homo Sapiens, is enough to explain the mystery of birth. But for the spiritual aspirant there is an understanding that all physical laws are merely reflections of deeper spiritual laws. And that it is in the understanding and attunement to these higher principles that we will find freedom from the limitations of the physical body and the fulfillment of the soul's natural desire to live in harmony with Spirit.

By connecting our view of life to the universal forces that have brought the creation into existence we can begin to understand the purpose of life. Once that purpose is perceived we can then step forward to help or hinder the process as we choose.

In many ways life is like a magic trick; not understood until you begin to look at it from the magician's perspective. When we look at life from a universal point of view, rather than the limited view of the ego, we can begin to see that while life is "magical" in its wondrous nature, it is not unexplainable.

For centuries the science of yoga has presented a very clear description of the mechanics, or metaphysics, of the way the universe operates. It is important to understand that the truth of these principles is not based on Hinduism, Christianity or any other religion, but that all religions in the world are unified by these basic tenets. It is these underlying principles that we will be focusing on as we explore childbirth.

So take a deep breath and dive with me into very deep waters, where we will explore life's purpose and the way in which it manifests.

The continuation of the human species isn't just for the sake of the natural evolution of the planet that we call Earth. It is the process through which souls can incarnate into this school of spiritual evolution that is called life on the physical plane.

God's manifestation of the creation is an outpouring of consciousness that comes from an unmanifested state of infinite ever-new bliss. As that consciousness reaches out from the ocean of Spirit it first manifests as thought. It is those ideational principles that comprise what is known as the Causal Plane.

The Causal Plane, the universe of ideas or thoughts, provides the substructure from which the creation then continues its outward push into limitation. Connecting this Material Plane in which we live, to the Causal Plane of thought, is the Astral Plane of energy. The manifestation of thought as energy is the midway point in creation's outward journey from timeless Spirit. It is in the Astral Plane that souls live between earthly incarnations in physical form. For a more detailed look at the nature of the Astral and Causal worlds I refer you to Chapter 43 of *Autobiography of a Yogi* by Paramhansa Yogananda.

The ancient scriptures of India explain that the process of reincarnation is the way in which the soul has the opportunity to start fresh in each life – like coming into a new classroom at the start of a school year – so that we can more easily grow towards our reawakening into the soul's true nature as ever existing, ever conscious, ever-new joy.

The teaching of reincarnation isn't limited to the religions of the east. It is also found in Christianity. Jesus asked his disciples, "Who do people say that I am?" And they answered, "Some say you are Elisha and others say that you are Elijah." The doctrine of reincarnation was actually a part of the church dogma until it was removed by the Second Council of Constantinople in 553 A.D.

While a belief in reincarnation isn't necessary for spiritual growth, when considering the subject of childbirth it is helpful to realize that the soul is not the body. The soul is individualized Spirit which has only temporarily become identified with the body through the ego.

The reality of the soul's separateness from the body is becoming more and more a matter of proven clinical truth rather than what some would call spiritual speculation. A number of studies have been done with people who have clinically died on the operating table and then were revived, or were left for dead and reawakened on their own. The clear consistency of conscious experience during those periods of "deadness" is a mounting clinical proof of life after life.

My own father-in-law had such an experience after suffering a heart attack. His heart stopped for some time and while the doctors were reviving him he had an "out of body" experience in which he found himself in the presence of the most loving beings that he could ever have imagined. He then consciously returned to his body because he was told that it wasn't yet his time. Although he was very weak at the time he immediately called my wife Bhavani to his side so that he could relate his fantastic experience.

Positive Flow Childbirth

Even though he had never read anything about the studies being done on this subject, his description of what happened was totally consistent with the experiences of many others.

The important thing to remember, regardless of what spiritual tradition one follows, is that the birth of a soul into this world is not just a physical event. It is a special gift that has its purpose rooted in the very manifestation of the creation itself.

It is a quirk of this world that because most of our energies are directed outward we think that the solutions to life's challenges are outside of us, rather than inside of us. But the keys to higher perception lie within us. And so it is with a sense of inner understanding that we should approach our involvement with the emergence into this world of a soul.

Chapter 2

The Positive Flow

Underlying the many decisions that we have to make in our lives is the basic problem: How do I know what the right thing to do is? The conflict starts when we use our Western way of thinking, which says that there is only one right answer to any question. The act of looking at life from a black and white, right and wrong perspective, is the very thing that starts us off on the wrong foot.

Instead of thinking right or wrong it is helpful to see life as a flow. Making choices which flow towards a more perfect expression of Spirit are beneficial. Decisions that flow away from universal truth are not beneficial.

How do we know the difference?

Spirit flows naturally towards selflessness - which is positive and expansive. Any elevating quality that brings with it a sense of expansive harmony is in its nature that which will bring us closer to God. Selfish qualities contract the spirit. They create disharmony and separate us from our unity with life. Selfishness binds us to the ego. The ego is the soul identified with the body and the more identified with the body that we are the less we can perceive of our reality as expressions of Spirit.

For instance, when we give spontaneously out of the

joy of giving we are expanding our sympathies and joining in the positive flow of life. If we cut in line so that we can get our share before the supply runs out, then we are acting selfishly, which contracts the heart and cuts us off from the oneness of love that binds all mankind.

Most of our experiences are a mixture of these positive and negative impulses, like doing a good deed partly for the recognition and partly because it is a good thing to do. And of course, different actions have different levels of energy attached to them. Cutting in line with a friendly smile and explanation of the fact that you are really in a hurry isn't nearly as bad as having a fist fight over who will get the last free donut.

As we begin to look at our decisions from this more fluid perspective we begin to realize that God's Will for us in this world isn't always as specific as: Eat peas and not beans! Or, turn left and not right. There is more than one way to express the good in life.

While it is true that at some time we might feel inspired to act in a particular way, the majority of the decisions that we make in life can be more easily dealt with if we attune ourselves to the positive flow of the life that is always available to us. By making a habit of living in this flow our natural reaction to any given situation will be a reflection of that positive flow.

It is continuous, conscious effort to be "in tune" with the positive flow of life that will lead us to the goal of expressing intuitive, wisdom-guided will – which is God's, Will. When we act for ego gratification we are expressing selfish will. This contracting, limiting will cuts us off from our highest potential.

The soul's natural desire to expand fully into Infinite Spirit should be seen as the basis of God's Will for us. All of the experiences that we have in this life are opportunities to enter into that expanding process.

The Positive Flow

There are numerous ways to consciously develop our awareness of inner truth. Some techniques are designed for specific areas like: awakening the heart, developing intuitive wisdom or cultivating a serviceful attitude. Other techniques are for changing our consciousness on more global levels. The most central of the techniques that can transform the totality of our consciousness is the practice of meditation.

Keep in mind that meditation, in itself, is not associated with only one particular spiritual tradition. All of the major religions have taught some form of meditation. The key to understanding the real purpose of meditation is to look at what naturally happens to the soul along its journey to achieving union with the Divine.

From the lives of the saints of all religions we find common underlying truths that are not bound by outward traditions. In all cases, the ecstasy of the saints is marked by a withdrawal of the energy from the senses and the single pointed direction of the soul's essential life force inward and upward, towards the mid-point between the eyebrows. As Jesus said, "If thine eyes be single, thy whole body shall be filled with light."

It is this process of interiorization and single pointed concentration of the mind and will that is so important to spiritual perception. Meditation techniques are specifically designed to help us achieve this ability to withdraw our awareness from the senses and perceive truth directly.

Spiritual perceptions never come by accident. If we want to know truth we must activate the process by showing our interest. Through meditation we can directly experience Spirit as our most basic reality. It is only from that basis that we can then move towards true understanding in any aspect of our lives. It is also easy to see, as we will discuss later in more detail, that the ability to withdraw one's awareness from the senses will present some very interesting possibilities when those contractions start!

When trying to harmonize our lives with truth, self honesty is essential. This may not seem so important at this stage of our discussion but when we get into the various specific issues surrounding childbirth it will be easy to see that our desires – whether they be in relative terms good, bad or no big thing one way or the other – will have to be faced. Without a willingness to look at how we really feel we won't be able to focus our energies harmoniously into doing that which is right, regardless of how we feel about it. Remember, without a sense of harmony, we disconnect ourselves from higher truth.

There are many difficult decisions to make in life. When we feel the inner harmony that comes from the knowledge that we are acting in the best possible way, according to the highest truth that we can perceive, then no matter how difficult the challenge may be the powers of the universe will come to our side. For when we are acting as channels for the highest truth we are fulfilling in the best way our part of the creation and manifesting the will of our Creator.

Chapter 3

To Child
or
Not to Child?

There are few times in life when we know more clearly than with the birth of a child, exactly what God's purpose is in this world. That purpose is the pure and unencumbered expression of love. If we take the expansion of our human love towards infinite Divine Love as the goal of life, we can see the bond between parent and child as one of the most fertile grounds for developing the kind of love that has no limit.

The challenge of love doesn't come with the easy part; like loving a cuddly smiling baby. It comes with the tests of endurance to which every parent can bear witness – the nights without sleep, the days of constant giving, the all too often fluctuation between times of extreme exasperation and moments of incredible closeness. It is in the fire of life's moment by moment challenges that our love is tempered and strengthened.

Before we enter into the firmament of parenthood we would do well to reflect on our circumstances in life, for the responsibilities of parenthood will reach into every part of our existence. Take the time to evaluate how having a child will affect your relationship with your spouse. Look at your home life in general and your job. Think about the things that you do for recreation. Consider your finances and how having a child will affect them. What about the quiet time in your life that you cherish?

Don't be afraid to look at your health and your family history. There are many hereditary conditions that should be thoroughly researched before a decision is made. Many potential problems with the health of the fetus can be traced to heredity. Take the time to learn about your family medical history so that you don't overlook something obvious that can be a major factor in your health or the health of your child.

Mental health is also an issue that isn't looked at often enough. Sometimes people having a rough time in their life think that having a child will make things better. More often than not, it doesn't.

Take a long, serious look at all of the physical plane ramifications that you can think of. Read up to get some other ideas. Be willing to take a soul searching look at these issues, but don't let the scope of the task scare you off. All great rewards are preceded by prodigious efforts!

By looking at these easier-to-see physical realities we have begun to consciously attune ourselves to the energies surrounding childbirth. While considering all of these factors ask yourself inwardly, "How does this feel?" "How does that feel?" This process of attunement is at the very heart of the spiritual life.

In fact, attunement is a key factor for success in any endeavor. Some people are under the impression that trying to live spiritually is incapacitating when it comes to dealing with the practical side of life. But the truth is that when we attune ourselves to the source of life itself we have at our disposal the resources of the universe! What could be more practical than that?

How can we tap into those infinite resources?

Well, we start with common sense. We don't expect to eat the feast before we have prepared it. It is a spiritual truism that we should always have a positive attitude and expect the best in life. It is also a truism that we shouldn't presume on God's intercession.

If we start off on a three week trek across a desert with no water and presume that God will provide for us, in most cases we will be making a presumption that will lead to the end of a physical incarnation. Making conscious decisions and aligning them with the highest truth that we are able to honestly perceive is a guideline that we should use in our preparation process.

As I mentioned in the previous chapter, meditation is the soil in which we can grow the flowers of our inner realization. To the techniques of meditation I would also add prayer. Once the mind is calm and interiorized through meditation the will can be focused like a broadcasting station in order to create a magnetism that will draw a Divine response. Sometimes, depending on the strength of our call and the depth of our receptivity, a response is immediate. At other times we must wait for signs. The signs, which are a signal as to Gods Will for us can come in an infinite number of ways. As each person's special relationship with God is developed the channels through which God tries to speak to us become more and more clear.

The key is to include God in our decision making process. Ask Him/Her for guidance and then listen with a calm inner awareness for the Divine response. Practice freeing yourself from attachment to your desires in any given situation and let God's response have an open acceptance in your heart.

Wouldn't life be easier if every time we had a difficult decision to make the heavens would open up and - with

Positive Flow Childbirth

suitable fanfare! - a heavenly being would pronounce the will of God? Well, for better or for worse, it isn't often that easy. There are however times in our lives when we get a very close approximation to a heavenly edict. It may be without the fanfare, but once something has happened in our lives and we can't avoid it, then, whether we wanted it or not, we must deal with it. There is nothing more sure in life than the fact that God wants us to deal with our experiences in the very best way that we can. For it is in our reaction to all of life's circumstances that we are tested and found ready to move ahead or in need of more practice.

Everyone has to deal with the unexpected, but when it comes to having children it is immeasurably more practical, as well as spiritually beneficial, to think deeply about it first.

We shouldn't take lightly the responsibility of bringing a soul into this world. The soul as individualized spirit is by definition a part of God. As parents we will be the physical plane stewards of this expression of God. We are God's representatives in this world. We must do our best to be worthy of that trust.

By consciously and actively seeking to make positive choices in life we are sowing the seeds for success. Next, we have to water them!

Chapter 4

Doorway to a New Lifetime

Once we have felt the inner correctness of bringing a child into this world we can turn to the subject of how to do it in the best possible way. For many at this point thoughts are turned towards mad, passionate love-making. But for the spiritually inclined there is much to do before we get to the actual act.

The ancient scriptures of India describe birth into a physical form as a sacred gift from God. It is in this material world that we can most quickly move towards our goal of self-realization. The divine manifestation of the battling forces of light and dark in this world motivate us to push forward in our search for eternal happiness.

Let's take a metaphysical look at what happens at the time of conception.

In the Astral Plane there are many more souls seeking physical incarnation than there are human forms to receive them. Some souls want to incarnate so that they can again enjoy the outwardly stimulating pleasures of this world. Others may not want to come here at all but are forced to through the law of karma. More advanced souls seek incarnation because of the spiritual benefits for advancement. In any case, the shortage

Positive Flow Childbirth

of physical bodies makes a physical incarnation all the more valuable.

Life works in a more subtle way in the Astral Plane than it does in the Physical World. Instead of taking applications for physical birth and notifying the lucky winners by post, souls are drawn by magnetic attraction at the time of physical conception. It is said that there is an actual spark in the ether and souls who are attuned to that specific vibration are attracted. In some cases there is a mad dash: Winner take all!

The moment of conception is the actual doorway through which the soul becomes identified with the physical world. It is important to understand the nature of this entry into the physical form. The fact that souls are magnetically drawn to a particular vibration means that if we can affect the vibration at the time of conception, then we can affect the quality of the soul that we will draw into our family. This is why it is so important to properly prepare ourselves before conception. This preparation time is equally, if not more important, than the physical birth itself. For once a soul is attracted, that's it, and the details of how it will emerge into this world, while also important, are secondary.

Since soul attraction is based on vibration, we need to work directly with the quality of our own vibrations as a central starting point. This is equally important for both the man and the woman.

Daily meditation should be the foundation of our efforts to raise our energy level and power of positive attraction. If we do nothing else; we should meditate. This time spent each day in deep communion with the love, peace and joy of Spirit is the most positively transforming of all human activities. It will help attract to us souls that, like ourselves, are seeking to live in harmony with life's positive potential.

After you have calmed yourself in meditation call to God. Ask for attunement in this process and pray that the Divine Will be done. Then, with a sense of peaceful communion and positively activated will, broadcast your soul call to the Astral World. Feel your energy rising in the spine and shooting out your spiritual eye like a beacon. If you want to you can also raise your arms and feel the energy flowing out of your fingertips. Sometimes it helps if you rub your hands briskly together before raising them so you can more easily feel the energy.

Mentally send words of invitation or simply radiate your love. If you feel in tune with Eastern traditions you can chant AUM (sounds like OM) while you feel the universal AUM vibration flowing through you. Remember that the exact words or style you use are not as important as the quality of your efforts. The key is that you are acting consciously as a channel for God's Will to be done. You are awakening a powerful energy flow and just like an electromagnet you are increasing your magnetism. This attunement to God's flow is the most powerful way that we can raise our vibration and draw a compatible soul to us.

Once you feel a sense of inner attunement try to hold on to it by keeping your mind calm. The peaceful mind is like the still surface of a pond. If we throw pebbles of restless thoughts into the waters we will lose our peace.

Mental stimulants like most music, movies, television, recreational books and excessive talking should be restricted during this time of consciously trying to draw a soul to your family. Only do those things that bring you a greater sense of peacefulness. High action and horror movies should be carefully considered before being viewed. Uplifting books, including those about the lives of the saints, are an excellent source of inspiration.

Positive Flow Childbirth

Many people don't realize the strong effect music has on our inner consciousness. The saying that "You are what you eat!" can also be phrased, "You are what you listen to!" Listen only to music that uplifts your soul and brings you closer to Spirit.

While inner attunement also raises the vibration of our physical bodies, there are some physical things that we can do that will help as well. These are ideas that you will want to add to the routine of your life if they aren't already present. They will be helpful not only for drawing a spiritual soul, but for easing the birth process itself and for improving our lives in general.

Try to eat healthfully.

If you are already a vegetarian, great! Along with the general health benefits comes a more refined vibration. If you eat meat, try to eat less of it. Avoid beef and pork as much as possible; fish and fowl are much better. Fresh fruit, nuts, vegetables and whole grains are the most vibrationally uplifting foods, so include them in your diet as much as possible.

As with all areas of your life, use your common sense. Any changes in your eating habits would best be done on a gradual basis. You can use your local health food store as a resource for healthful dietary information, and of course, consult a physician if you have any special needs or areas of concern.

By no means am I saying that what you eat will in itself determine the soul that you will draw to yourself. But a healthful diet makes it easier for you to free yourself from body consciousness and that will help you raise your vibration.

Reduce the stress in your life!

Tensions that build up in the body and mind from a wide variety of sources in our lives make it much harder for us to feel the peace of Spirit. Look at your life in general and try to avoid or minimize things that cause you stress. Do what you can to counterbalance stresses that you can't avoid. Get plenty of exercise. Try to spend time out in nature. Smile regularly!

Have you ever tried a class in Hatha Yoga? It is a system of body positions that are designed to release mental and physical stress. They are also a perfect preparation for meditation. In fact, that is what they were original created for, a system for preparing the body and mind for inner communion with Spirit.

These are just some of the ways to keep the body and mind fit for expressing the joys of Spirit and for positively magnetizing your life. Use your own divinely guided creativity in coming up with more ways that work for you.

Try to spend three to six months giving special attention to your efforts in drawing the right soul for your family. A year wouldn't be too long and even a day would be better than none. Some people shop for days, even months, just to find the right dress, hat, car or house. Let's give at least equal attention to drawing the right soul into our family.

Make the power of your magnetic call strong so that the right soul won't be able to resist your loving invitation.

Chapter 5

Choosing a Time

When trying to choose the right time to have a child there are things that we can easily point to and say, "I would prefer that." Then there are issues that will take much time and thought. But beware! There are also things that will come up unexpectedly and say, "Change in plans ahead!"

Try to remember the flow as we make logical decisions. Let your positive flow of inner knowing be the force that pulls all of the possibilities together for you. When you don't feel attunement to the positive flow, take the time to meditate.

Let's look at a few factors just to get your own ideas flowing. If you want, make a list of more considerations as they occur to you. Evaluate each one by itself and then in combination with others. You might try listing each area according to its flexibility. Use labels like: can't change, hard to change, easy to change, no big deal, and maybe, want to change!

It can be helpful in your planning process to look at the calendar. There are a wide variety of subjects that can be discussed when considering the time of year. List things like a yearly convention that Dad just can't afford to miss. If Mom is working, she probably doesn't want to be in her third trimester during the busiest time of the year. What about having the baby during vacation time so that Dad can stay home for a while after the birth? If Mom or Dad are teachers, then maybe during summer when school is out would be the best time. Will your business health insurance cover the costs if you wait a while? What else?

Social calendars should also be considered. Do you always go somewhere for a particular holiday each year? Is there a summer camping trip that you would hate to miss? What about an anniversary getaway that you promised yourselves always to take? Can you think of any other date that might be an issue?

Look at other areas in your life that will be affected, like educational, vocational or financial goals. Maybe you want to travel before parenting? Weather can even be a factor. Do you live in a rural area where it snows? Keep thinking! Be honest and complete in your exploration of these ideas. You may decide to put off having a child for some time. That would be better than wishing you had waited, when it's too late!

The point of looking at these issues isn't that any one factor is more important than the birth of your child or that you will absolutely be able to avoid a trouble area. The goal is to let yourself enjoy visualizing the possibilities and maybe in the process save yourself a lot of unexpected and unnecessary grief. Taking the time to look at these considerations is part of what takes us out of the "Oh let's make a baby today!" or "Oops, we made a baby!" attitudes which have torn many families asunder.

As you make your way through this process always try to maintain your sense of God's active presence in your deliberations. This is what turns us towards acting responsibly in the highest sense of the word.

There is another aspect of timing that is much more subtle and yet has a very strong effect on us. Our world, as a manifestation of thought - which has become solidified by its coverings of energy and then matter - is in itself a kind of magnet. It is said that only souls that are in tune with this particular world's magnetism are drawn here.

Just as souls evolve, so do worlds. The magnetic influences of the universe have an ongoing effect on our world as each day goes by. The actual time and place that a soul is born into this world has a subtle magnetic imprint from these universal forces. This imprint is the basis of the science of astrology.

I am not referring to the shallow outward predictions that you read in many daily newspapers, but to a much more subtle and spiritual understanding of astrology. If you have never delved into this area before because of the superficiality of what you have seen, you might consider getting a good book on the subject. Preferably one that emphasizes the spiritual aspects of astrology. It isn't for everyone, and it certainly isn't essential, but it is worthy of consideration.

Regardless of whether you feel inclined to consider any astrological factors, remember, the soul is at anytime free through the application of will to overcome outward influences. By developing our inner strength through spiritual practices we are able to counterbalance negative influences and to align ourselves with positive influences.

Once you have ascertained the best time of the year for the birth then all you have to do is count back to the appropriate date for conception. Easy, right? Well, as we all know, life has a way of being unpredictable just when we think we have a handle on it. There are a number of foreseeable and unforeseeable things that can throw off your calculations.

While, for the sake of family planning, the avoidance of teenage pregnancy and other health considerations, it is often discussed how easy it is to become pregnant, the fact is it doesn't always happen the first time you try. So you might have to factor this into your plans. Study some material on the fertility cycle if you want to get as much control over the date of the birth as possible. If you start to feel that conception isn't happening as it should, consult a physician. Difficulties in conceiving a child are not all that uncommon, so you shouldn't see such difficulties, in themselves, as a sign that you aren't supposed to have children.

But as always, be open to the flow that God has for you. If you are having a problem it may be so that you can manifest the will to overcome it. It may also be a sign to stop and reevaluate your circumstances. A deeply personal situation like this takes the mustering of your spiritual strength and the melting away of your desires into a sense of harmony with God's Will. As the challenges present themselves take them one by one. Take courage from your knowledge that all of the experiences that we have in life are designed to give us opportunities to come closer to God.

For most couples conception won't be a physiological problem, so as we have discussed, take the time to plan things out. Have fun with it! And keep praying for guidance and attunement so that your decisions will be in tune with God's highest flow for you.

Chapter 6

Gathering Your Forces

One of the most basic challenges for the spiritual aspirant is that we have trouble focusing our energies single-pointedly on our goal. Our thoughts and actions are scattered in such a way as to diminish our ability to awaken our inner resources and concentrate them fully. Let's talk about some of the things that we can do to gather and focus our inner resources.

One of the things that we can do for both physical and spiritual benefit is to abstain from intercourse for a period of time before trying to conceive. It is a time for gathering and magnetizing our forces; especially for the man. The semen is a physical manifestation of the vital life force that resides in an astral vortex at the base of the spine. While this energy is present in both men and women, it is much stronger in men; as evidenced by their generally stronger sex drive.

The value of storing these vital energies is that it increases one's inner strength, and thus, one's magnetism. The power of this magnetism can be applied to both material as well as spiritual objectives. It is a powerful force that if used wisely can make the difference between average or great success in life. If that energy is used in an effort to elevate one's vibration and draw a sensitive soul, instead of just the enjoyment of a sexual relationship, then much can be achieved toward our goal of attracting a compatible soul to our family.

How long should you abstain from intercourse? There is no exact amount of time. On one side we find the rare person who is honestly comfortable living a celibate life unless trying conceive a child. On the other side we find most of the human race! As when evaluating much of what we face in life, choose a starting point and look at it honestly. Can you live with it? Could you handle more? Will it cause you to go absolutely crazy?

One thought is to make this period of time long enough that it will be personally challenging without going past the point of diminishing returns. Both partners should look within themselves along with discussing it together. Remember, the decision making process and the resolution should bring increased harmony to your relationship. For if you lose your harmony, then much if not all of the value of abstinence will be lost.

Along with sexual abstinence should come a general pulling in of your commitments to outward activity. It isn't necessary that you become a recluse, but more time spent alone with God is always beneficial.

This idea of gathering your forces is a balance between not wasting energies on one hand and increasing them through wholesome Spirit reminding activities on the other hand. Activities that are in tune with the positive flow of life actually give us more energy because we get used to larger and larger amounts of energy flowing through our lives.

While it is true that the body does store energy, the body is not in essence a storage battery. It is a conduit. The more we perceive God's energy flowing through us the more we connect to the unlimited life force that is always available to us.

Positive Flow Childbirth

All we need to do is tap into it and then learn how to channel it. That is how the Saints perform miracles. They have learned to channel the power of the universe through the conduit of their consciousness. By removing any ego desire they naturally manifest the Divine Will without the physical limitations to which we have become accustomed.

Remember when we talked about the Causal World and how it is based on thought? Those thoughts are consciousness. Our own lives are activated by the flow of Divine consciousness. Tuning in to this inner flow of consciousness is the central solution to all of life's challenges. Even for conceiving a child.

So don't take lightly this idea of gathering your forces. It can bring amazing results.

Chapter 7

The Spiritual Nature of Sexuality

Sexuality is a very difficult subject for many people to talk about. When you mix a wide range of social and religious taboos with a world that uses sexuality to advertise almost every type of product, what is a person to think? Can sexuality even be connected to spirituality?

Let's start by remembering that God made the creation. As the Mother/Father of life, God certainly knows all about what is going on! Not only that, but God is the creation. So let's throw away all embarrassment and discomfort. While God's creation might seem quite bizarre at times, it is also incredibly beautiful. When we begin to see life's drama as an expression and a part of God then we can see more clearly what our part in life is all about.

As we've discussed, in order to manifest the creation God had to express out of the infinite void a stream of consciousness. It went out from the unlimited infinite bliss of spirit towards the limited expression of spirit that we call the creation. That stream of consciousness first left infinite understanding to become limited thought. Then it coalesced as energy and finally, at its farthest point became clothed as the world of matter.

Positive Flow Childbirth

This outward flow of life is the male principle. It is the "Let's get out there and do it!" drive that keeps the creation going. Without it the creation would stop manifesting itself.

The male sexual organs are outside of the body. This is an example of how the underlying universal principles of life are outwardly manifested in the physical world. The male drive for procreation in all species is compelled by this inner force: the Divine Will to perpetuate the creation.

Just like a wave that has crested high above the ocean, the creation after it has reached its farthest point away from its beginning in unmanifested Spirit, starts the long inward journey home. This is the female principle, the divine flow back towards our state of rest in the bosom of Spirit.

The female sexual organs are within the body, hinting at the inward direction that we must go to reunite with Spirit. Also showing the importance of receptivity as a balance to the male drive for action. The female breasts are found outside of the body. This represents the giving, loving nature that reaches out as a natural expression of the soul as it reflects the ever-nurturing Divine Mother.

By looking at these causative forces we begin to see that sexuality is, at its very root, based on the creative principles of life itself. All of life in large and small rhythms and cycles pulses with this dance of the inward and outward – that which flows towards infinite Spirit and that which flows toward material world limitation.

In India these forces are called Prakriti and Aprakriti. In the Orient it is known as Yin and Yang. This is why we live in a world of duality: positive and negative, hot and cold, pleasure and pain. Each life experience has a corresponding opposite. These universal principles need to be understood if we want to put, not only our sexuality, but all of our motivating forces into a perspective that really makes sense. When we live in the positive expanding energy that is flowing toward infinite Spirit we are living in the positive flow of life. When we live in the contracting energy of life that is flowing toward limitation we are living in the negative flow of life.

We need to realize that each of us has accumulated our own unique mixture of energies during our long journey through the creation. This accumulation of energies is called Samskara - the sum total of our karma which covers the soul. The soul itself is neither male nor female. When we incarnate into a new body, according to our karma from the past, we may be born sometimes in a male body and sometimes in a female body.

The thought of having been in the past a gender opposite to which we are now experiencing might at first be disturbing. But as we ponder the many mixtures of impulses that people experience this idea explains much. Isn't it true that some men by their loving nurturing nature seem more feminine than many women? Aren't some women as tough and brash as any man can be? To explain this variety of expressions simply by discussing hormones is to divorce ourselves from the larger realities of life. And that, by definition, is what the negative flow of life tries to do to us. It tries to convince us that limited matter and not unlimited Spirit is the basis of life.

The mixtures of energies that we feel within us are the result of the spiritual law of karma. Karma means action. We carry within us the seeds of all our past actions. This activating principle is outwardly expressed by the law of physics that says: For every action there is an equal and opposite reaction. Some simply say, "What goes around comes around."

The idea is that when we act, be it in thought or deed, we will receive the fruits of those actions. If we act unkindly towards others we will draw unkindness to ourselves. If we are giving by nature, then we will receive giving energy.

The universal magnetic reaction to our actions is always balanced and equal to the energies that we radiate from within. But when you consider the incredible mixture of energies that each individual soul carries from many incarnations, added together with the energies of all other souls, plus planetary and universal influences, it's hard to believe at times that it is all going to balance out in the end.

Fortunately, this incredible complexity can be simplified by our understanding of the positive flow of life towards Spirit. When we live in that flow two very important things start to happen. The first is that we stop adding to the list of negative actions that we have already done. The second is that we begin to neutralize all of our negatively charged energies from the past by adding to the power of our positively charged energies. Thankfully, when we create a strong positive force in our lives we are much less affected by the negative energies that we created in the past.

The sum total of these positive and negative energies defines our vibration. To raise our vibration, instead of trying to dig out each little problem of the past and facing it alone, mano a mano, like many psychologists would recommend, we create a powerful positive spiritual force within us through meditation and attunement to the positive flow in life. Then with the application of sufficient will we can achieve any goal to which we apply ourselves.

I should mention that there are times when it can be helpful to use traditional psychological techniques for dealing with individual problems. Many of life's challenges, including but not limited to different mental illnesses, need professional psychological attention. But these services are usually pointed at the solving of one or at best a few of our challenges. The techniques of the spiritual life will in the long run resolve all of our challenges.

In order to help this process of soul evolution we need to act in ways that don't bind us to our actions. This is called Nishkam-Karma, desireless action. These are actions done without the desire for the fruits of our actions. When we act in accordance with the laws of truth and align ourselves with life's positive flow, then we begin to feel that it isn't the little self of ego acting but the larger Self of Spirit acting through this particular channel. Then we can begin to act with the knowledge that God is living through us, that His power animates us, and that He is in truth the doer of all things.

From this larger view we can see that our human sexuality is animated by the most elemental powers in the creation. The key to using it for our spiritual growth is to transform it from a chain that can bind us to the limited world of the senses into a powerful force that can bring us quickly to God. This can be so beautifully seen in the lives of the saints. While each has their own particular expression the common underlying presence of strength and love are undeniable. With the blending of the male and female principles we find a balance that can fully expresses the Divine.

Chapter 8

Transmuting Sexual Energy

Many people are under the mistaken impression that there is a spiritual injunction against participating in sexual activities. Actually, the sexual drive is one of the strongest powers that we can bring to bear towards our spiritual development, but it can also be our greatest downfall.

The issue, like so many others, isn't whether or not it should be a part of our lives: it is and there is no way around that. The key is what do we do with it? Do we use it to help us towards the achievement of our spiritual goals or do we let it keep us bound ever more firmly to the limited world of the senses?

Well, there is good news and bad news. Here's the scoop!

Thousands of years ago the yogis of India investigated this subject to the Nth degree. A well known volume called the *Kama Sutra* or "Verses of Love" is filled with much information on this subject. They found that you can actually use sexuality and sensuality in general as a path to self-realization. This is part of what is called the path of Tantric Yoga. The only problem with this path is that it is very, very difficult. Here is some background information so that you can understand the dilemma and decide how to deal with these issues in your own life.

The energy that animates us, called cosmic energy, enters the human form through the medulla oblongata. When the sperm and ovum unite at conception those two cells that have become one start to multiply. They first form the medulla which is at the base of the brain. The brain and then the rest of the body grow around the medulla.

Although we do get some of our energy from the combination of food and air, why is it that when someone dies we don't just feed and air them? Well, in fact, that is what doctors try to do when someone dies. They ventilate with oxygen and feed them different stimulating drugs. They even try to jump start the system with electricity. Sometimes their efforts are successful and at other times they aren't.

Why doesn't this type of resuscitation always work? Because once our life force is fully withdrawn from the body death is the result. In cases where people's bodies are "restarted" it means that their soul's life force was not fully disconnected.

It is the animating cosmic life force that actually causes the breath to flow and holds body and soul together. Without that life sustaining force we withdraw to the Astral World. From the medulla, through subtle nerve and astral channels, this life force is sent to seven distribution areas called Chakras. It is through these subtle centers of energy that the body's ability to function is animated, thus causing the many complex physiological systems to do their job.

Again, this is a case of looking at the underlying spiritual energies that cause physical plane laws to operate. These energy distribution centers are located along the center of the body just in front of the physical spine. Starting at the base of the spine is the coccyx center; a few inches up from there is the sacral center; then the lumbar center at the navel; the heart center; and the cervical center at the throat. The sixth center is at the medulla, but it has its positive pole at the spiritual eye - between and just above the eyebrows. The seventh center is called the thousand-petaled lotus and is located at the top of the head.

Connecting these seven chakras are two subtle channels called the ida and pingala. It is the flow of energy up and down the ida and pingala, on the left and right sides of the spine, that cause the breath to flow. There is also an even more subtle channel connecting the chakras called the sushumna. This is called the deep spine, located in the very center of the body and running from the coccyx center all the way up to the top of the head.

Whole treatises have been written on what we just covered in a few paragraphs so obviously there is much more that could be said. I am hoping you have gotten enough of a "lay of the land" so that the rest of our discussion on this subject makes some sense.

It is in these chakras that I have just described that all of our past karma is stored – vortices of energy, waiting dormant until the right outside influence comes along to activate it, and then, poof! It's payback time. Hopefully we have stored more pleasant karma than unpleasant!

When our life energy arrives at the chakras it has two paths that it can follow: out to the physical body and the senses or within towards the sushumna. When we direct our energies outward we become more sense conscious. Through the senses our energy is dissipated. The more it is dissipated the more we try to get it back by indulging the senses.

For most people the indulgence in sexual pleasure is simply that, indulgence in pleasure for the sake of pleasure. But what is the result? A cutting off from the only really soul-satisfying pleasure in the universe – the joy of Spirit. But, you say, I said there was a way to use the sexual energy to find God!

Okay here it is.

If the energy that we use to animate the senses is turned back toward the chakras, instead of out through the senses, then we can increase the flow of energy in the spine. Instead of dissipating it out through the senses we use it to awaken our spiritual awareness.

Let's try it again. If the energy that we feel in the senses is directed inward towards the spine and upward towards the brain, then we increase the inner energy with which we can perceive Spirit, instead of dissipating it through the senses.

This works with all of the senses. Let's use touch as an example. Your hand is rubbed and it feels good. If you are only aware of the pleasant effects of being touched than the energy of the experience is being dissipated and you are engrossed in limited sense awareness. Conversely, if you let the energy that you feel on your skin flow inside you, up your arm to the spine and then direct it up to the brain you are transmuting the sensual energy into upward flowing spiritual energy. The key is to keep the energy flowing into the spine and up towards the spiritual eye.

This is something that takes much practice to accomplish. The mind and emotions want to indulge in the pleasant touching while the soul wants to be detached from the limited senses and to rise within. It is a mighty struggle. And if you think to continually indulge in the senses under the mistaken idea that you are "transmuting the energy", then you can get pulled far down into a quagmire of sensuality which inevitably leads to suffering. Remember, when we live in the senses, for every pleasure there will be at some point and equal and opposite pain. That is the way this world of duality is made.

Positive Flow Childbirth

To make the idea of using sex to increase our inner connection to Spirit even more enticing, there is at the base of the spine a great power that is sleeping untapped. It is called the Kundalini energy or the serpent power. This dormant until awakened energy is so powerful that it can hurl our consciousness into very high states of awareness. It also activates the amazing powers that are available to the saints that produce what we call miracles.

Normally this Kundalini energy is awakened at a gradual pace and that is best. If it is activated too soon and we are not sufficiently able to control the energy properly, then we can find ourselves worse off than before it was awakened. The reason sexuality is often associated with the Kundalini power is that sexual energy is much stronger than any of the senses by themselves. So if you use sexuality to awaken the Kundalini it can potentially be accomplished more quickly.

Let me say clearly: The risks of overindulgence in sexuality and sense pleasures for the purposes of awakening the Kundalini far outweigh the potential benefits for 99.9% of us. The best course of action concerning sexuality and the senses in general is summed up in this truism: The senses never fed are ever satisfied and the senses ever fed are never satisfied. Think about it!

As always, moderation is a good rule of thumb and leaning towards less rather than more is even better. But, since we do live in a world in which we will be bombarded with sense input whether we want it or not, always try to transmute that which you perceive through the senses by drawing the energy into the spine and up to the spiritual eye.

Live more and more in the spine. Let your awareness of life radiate from the spiritual eye. Try always to be centered in your inner chamber of spiritual peace. As you develop your ability to meditate and practice living in the positive flow of life your inner energies will naturally in their own time awaken.

So for now, let the serpent sleep.

Chapter 9

Spiritualizing Physical Union

The pure desire for a man and a woman to express their love in physical union is a manifestation of the soul's desire to merge into Infinite Spirit and so it is with this consciousness of merging that we should approach the physical act of love-making. Many would agree that the act of sacrificing one's life for another is one of the greatest acts of giving that one can express in this world. The act of coming together in love, to bring a child into this world, is in its own way a similarly holy act. The soul's comings and goings from this world are times of great energy. This energy can be used to propel us forward towards greater spiritual awareness or it can hold us back.

As we come to the time of physical union let us keep in mind the sacred responsibility that we are accepting. This child will be a spark of God clothed in the form of a child. As parents we should see ourselves as divine representatives and do our very best.

Consider where your union will take place. You may want to go somewhere special or you may want to remain at home. Remember, the environment that you choose will affect you. Is it uplifting or downward pulling? Is it agitating or serene? As an example, an environment that is close to nature is more likely to be a calm and uplifting setting as compared to the restlessness of sense indulgence that you find in many adult focused resorts. The environment you choose can have an effect on the soul that you draw.

Prepare yourselves by being apart for a while. Time alone will help you to clarify and focus your energies. Spend this time meditating and inwardly attuning yourselves. Be as quiet as you can and let the peace of Spirit permeate your consciousness. It can also be helpful if you refrain from eating for at least three hours – longer would be good. Drink liquids according to your bodies needs, but don't fast to the point that you become light-headed. Let common sense guide you.

Bathing can also be given special attention. You can use a sauna or hot tub if you want. Water is calming to both body and mind. As you bathe feel that you are also washing away negative and restless thoughts. You can bath together if you choose, but don't let your intimacy cause you to jump the gun!

When deciding where you want to come together be sure that it will be comfortable and private! For many the bedroom is the place of choice. But there are no strict rules here, except that the environment enhance your closeness to Spirit and to each other. For some the woods or a secluded beach would be perfect, or a cabin in the mountains might be nice. One of the advantages of staying at home is that your vibrations are generally strongest there. But there also may be disadvantages to where you live: like people, noises, distractions and other disturbances. If you feel you won't be able to relax and concentrate at home then plan to go elsewhere.

Wherever you go, or if you stay at home, prepare the space and make it especially beautiful with flowers and/ or candles. If you feel to, spiritualize the space with pictures of the saints, incense and other holy objects that your revere.

Positive Flow Childbirth

If you plan on having music playing be sure that it is calming and inwardly focusing. You don't want to be drawn outside of yourself by the music.

The time of day or night that you choose should be balanced with your need for preparation time. One thing to keep in mind is that you don't want to be overly tired. Make it a time when you have sufficient energy to give it your full attention.

Now that everything is in place and you have prepared yourselves on your own inwardly and outwardly, spend some time together in meditation. Let your separate energies merge into the joy of Spirit. How long you meditate is up to you, but I would caution against going so long that your energy lags. As a general guideline I would recommend one half to two thirds of your regular meditation duration. If you are not a regular meditator than I would say ten to fifteen minutes. Be sure to pray for attunement and God's blessings.

If you have decided to create a ceremony of any kind or even with your prayers and meditation, try not to be too solemn. Stay relaxed, joyous and natural, for spontaneous lightness of heart is certainly one of God's ways of being with us in this world.

When you have finished your devotions come together with the inward joy that you feel in meditation. Let the love that you have connected to in Spirit flow through you to your partner, who is in essence a part of God. Fully appreciate the loving embrace in which you are now enveloped. Don't worry about whether you are transmuting your sexual energies, just let your experience flow from your heart and feel that you are offering yourself to the indwelling Spirit.

While you should fully enter into the inward and outward enjoyment of this time, don't let your mind be pulled into thoughts of lust. Keep the radiance of your love shining so brightly that lesser thoughts cannot enter.

The love that I am speaking of is not the kind of emotion that turns into passion, that kind of love is contracting and limited. Divine Love is always expanding and inclusive of others. It is giving and there is an unlimited abundance of it. This heavenly love is not something that we can hold; it is a power that flows through us. Feel it spreading out from your heart center and filling your whole being, then continue to expand that love so that you and your partner merge into the oneness of infinite love.

Whew!

When you are done – I won't presume to tell you how long to stay at it – try to stay enveloped in that sense of inner communion. Remember, you aren't really done yet, conception won't happen for some time. What you have done is plant the seeds and water them with God's love through you. Now as the laws of nature do their part, a soul is waiting in the wings to join your family. Stay inwardly calm and mentally broadcast your invitation to a compatible soul. The astral doorway will soon be opening!

Chapter 10

Conscious Conception

Receptivity is one of the key qualities in the spiritual life. Opening ourselves in humbleness to receive God's blessings is essential. As it says in the Bible, "To as many as received Him gave He the power to become the sons of God." The conception of a child is certainly one of God's blessings.

There are times in life when we somehow know within ourselves that great forces are at work. We may not be able to see them but our inward knowing tells us it must be so. This is such a time. The gap between the astral and physical worlds is going to be breached and into this world is going to come a soul who will be drawn here to continue their journey toward self-realization.

Your openness is now of great importance. As the time of conception comes near do your best to maintain a sense of inwardness. If you can spend time alone during this period, all the better. Not speaking to much or not at all helps to calm the mind. Many people don't realize how much energy is expended in idle chatter.

Physiologically it can be hours or days after intercourse before conception takes place. So, depending on your life's circumstances, you may or may not have a choice as to how you will spend that time. Here are some thoughts that can help both now and at any time you want to make special efforts to maintain an inward awareness.

To begin with, let's review what it is about any activity that causes it to be helpful or harmful to our level of awareness. When the mind is calm it is like a still pool of water. If we imagine the moon shining from above we can see its perfect reflection in the water. As long as the mind is calm it can perceive the subtle rays of spiritual perception that are always shining upon us from within.

Let's take that same calm pool and throw a pebble into it. What happens? Ripples! What do they do to our image of the moon? It isn't so easy to see now. Imagine throwing in thousands of pebbles. It would be a veritable storm of activity. Seeing the moon's reflection would become very difficult and the parts that you could see would be very fragmented. This is what happens in our minds as we receive all of the countless sensory stimuli that each day brings. Our minds become filled with impression upon impression, all bumping into each other in an endless stream of input. That's one of the causes of restless dreams. The subconscious mind has to sort out all of this input so that it can be ready for the next day.

There are a number of ways that we can deal with the input that we receive each day so that we don't lose our peace of mind and calmness of soul. The first thing to consider is environment. Try simply to avoid things and places that are excessively agitating. Loud noises, bright lights, quickly moving objects, loud and/or fast music, lots of people, these are all strong stimulants that can cause the mind to lose its peace.

Of course, just about every place on the planet has some of these things, it's the nature of the physical world. But there is a big difference between sliding down a slide at the

Positive Flow Childbirth

local park and riding a hundred foot tall roller-coaster. Sure, you might want to go to an amusement park once in a while, but not on a day to day basis. Yet, every day when we add up all of the stimulation from television, radio, billboards, travel time in the car, interactions with people, problems with this or that, all of life itself begins to look like an amusement park! It's not that any of these things are necessarily bad by themselves, but added up all together they cause us to become more sense oriented, rather than spirit oriented.

Will we live our lives in harmony or disharmony? This choice is made each day as we go through life and decide what we are going to do or how we are going to react to any given situation. If we want to choose harmony, peace and closeness to God, then we will need to find those qualities within ourselves and minimize our exposure and/or negative reaction to agitating outside influences.

While avoidance is one side of the equation, the other side is what we can do positively to increase our inner strength so that we are less affected by things that we can't avoid. This brings us back to the spiritual basics: meditation, prayer and aligning our lives with the positive flow of life. When we are firmly rooted in the peace of Spirit the problems of daily life have a much more difficult time throwing us off balance. By strengthening the good in our lives we are less affected by the negative.

One of the things that mothers can try to do is to actually be aware of the soul being drawn within you at the time of conception. It is an amazing thought, but it is quite possible. My wife at the time, Bhavani, was out in the garden planting some flowers when she felt a large surge of energy within herself. In that moment she intuitively recognized that conception had just occurred. She said that it was a little confusing because she

48

felt so much more energy than she had with either of her first two children from a previous marriage. Months later we found out why she had this difference of inner feeling. It wasn't just because Bhavani was more sensitive to the energies within her than she had been years earlier, it was because this time there were two souls: twins!

This idea of consciously greeting your child is certainly possible, although not easy. It takes a deep level of calmness and attentiveness. If you sensitize your awareness through the dedicated immersion in your spiritual practices and stay attentive you may be able to consciously greet your child. But even if you don't feel a soul entering your womb, immerse your thoughts in loving greeting during this time because there may be a soul inside you that has just been sucked out of the astral realm into a very confining body and it just might need a little loving!

Chapter 11

Soul Within a Soul

Have you ever wondered why mothers get so crazy while they are pregnant? Many women experience strange urges, unpredictable mood swings, endless hunger or a repulsion from food, the desire to be touched more or not at all, the list of possibilities is endless. Add to that list: aches and pains, swollen this or that, added weight and always needing to go to the bathroom. What's this commotion all about?

The traditional view of all this hoopla in the body is strictly physical. The body is being taken over by the gestation process and the appropriate hormones are doing their chosen tasks. From the "outside in" this explanation makes sense. We can capture this process on film and record it. Our minds can put the pieces together and deal with the results. Aren't we happy!?

For most people, that is where things stay, in the physical. And I certainly don't discount that this traditional view is part of the truth. But, as we have been discussing, by understanding the underlying spiritual forces that are always activating the life that we live we can use this greater understanding to our benefit. There is nothing more practical than learning to live in harmony with the forces that activate what we call nature.

Soul Within a Soul

As we look at this situation the first thing to remember is that a soul, with all of its attendant seeds of past karma and the energies associated with them, has just entered into the very depths of the mother's energies. The magnetic fields of mother and child are now intermingled. This unique relationship is part of what impresses the mother/child bond so powerfully. It can also make the mother go a little nuts! Suddenly there are new and strange impulses inside the mother that she has never had before. As the child's soul identifies more and more with this new body and circumstance it starts to put energy into its own view of the way things should be. This blending of physical, mental and emotional energies is so disorienting at times that it is enough to make you feel like throwing up – as so many mothers do!

Even though the child is yet unborn outside of the mother's body, conception is when parenting for a specific soul actually starts! As a parent your responsibility is to love and nurture the soul that has taken up temporary residence within you. It doesn't really matter if you feel physically good or bad, the child must be nurtured. So start to consciously communicate with and love your child from day one in the womb.

The amazing thing is that this process of conscious attunement not only enhances one's good feelings about what is taking place but the child responds to the loving, caring thoughts that you are sending. And so does the rest of your body. Mothers who feel this attunement generally have fewer physical problems and are better able to deal with the ones that they do have.

Too many mothers try to fight the conflicting energies that they are feeling. It seems like a war going on inside and they are determined to win. But the way to win the tug-of war with this child's energy is not to fight it but to harmonize with it.

51

Positive Flow Childbirth

Try to open yourself up to what the child is feeling or needing. Listen carefully for silent whispers of communication that might be coming your way.

Let's look at it from the baby's point of view for a minute. Unless it is a very high soul, it may not be sure what is going on. Having been drawn out of the astral world, probably not of its own volition, it has also left behind memory of past lives. Those rare souls that have fully realized their oneness with Spirit and are returning to this earth to bless mankind are totally aware of all that is happening during this time if they choose to be.

On the other end of the spectrum are souls that have very limited perceptions and are basically asleep for their nine month stay in the womb. Most souls are in the middle somewhere and are capable of varying degrees of awareness. Of course as time goes by they become more and more identified with this new body. Like anything new, it takes some getting used to. The kicking and moving around that takes place in the womb isn't just muscular spasms caused by hormones, but an exploration of this new form by the soul.

As with all relationships, communication is the key. It should be heartfelt and two way. Since the child can't speak to you verbally you will need to listen for thoughts that weren't in your mind before. They may or may not be consciously directed toward you by your new family member. Knowing your inner self very well before conception will make you better prepared to recognize these subtle changes in your consciousness.

Expressing an attitude that reflects complete harmony with Spirit in all of life's circumstances is certainly one of the graces of self-realization. Along the way to that goal we sometimes have to take on an attitude that we know is correct, even though we don't immediately feel in tune with it. What happens is that by practicing attitudes which express harmony with the positive flow of life and not giving in to attitudes that express the negative flow of life we strengthen our natural inclination to do the right thing.

I'm not saying that we should suppress our feelings. What we need to do is transmute them in just the same way that we talked about with the senses. Instead of letting the energy dissipate in emotional outbursts - be they happy or sad - we can transmute them into attunement with the positive flow. When you are feeling down: affirm joy! When you feel restless: affirm peace! When you are flying too high: affirm calmness!

Certainly it takes some practice to turn negative energies towards positive directions, but it is eminently worth the effort. Keep in mind that when we make an effort to attune ourselves to the positive flow of life, that positive flow meets us more than half way. So the distance to our positive goals in life aren't always as far away as they may seem.

During the pregnancy, try to stay a little detached from your mood swings. Let your goal be to maintain a sense of even-mindedness and cheerfulness. With the swirling energies due to the excitement of being pregnant, the child's energies within - and yes, don't leave out those busy little hormones! - it is easy to lose control of emotions. While it is natural to be excited, beware of extremes. By mentally standing back a little you will be able to see with some impartiality what is going on in the mental and emotional landscape of your mind.

If you find yourself swinging too far one way or the other, redirect your attention by putting your energy strongly in a positive direction. This could be meditation, yoga postures, taking a walk, doing a hobby, reading a book, taking a bath or visiting with a friend. Anything that redirects your energy in a positively calming way.

Positive Flow Childbirth

Along with your attempts to stay detached and even-minded, cultivate the attitude of patience. Don't be too hard on yourself. I'm not suggesting that you should indulge yourself in every little whim, but if you get ruffled now and again don't add to it by lingering on it. Move on towards all of the positive things in your life.

Many women are very physically self-conscious while they are carrying a child. The body is going through massive changes, it is normal and healthy to put on some weight. Sometimes women feel that these changes make them less attractive. Have you ever noticed that at special times in a person's life they seem to be aglow with some special radiance? This emanation from within can be seen most easily as joy shinning through the eyes and love radiating from the heart. This inner glow is a reflection of the infinite potential that we all have within our souls. Mothers to be always shine with that glow and it is more beautiful than all of the diamonds in the world, or a slim figure! All mothers are a part of God fulfilling one of the most beautiful of human roles. So do your best to stay healthy and don't sweat the details!

At this stage your child will already have begun imprinting patterns that they will carry all the way through this new lifetime. Help make those patterns as spiritual as possible. One of the greatest blessings that you can give your child at any time, but especially in the womb, is the feeling of God's presence. During this commingling of spirits try to immerse yourself and your child in the love, joy and peace of Spirit.

Chapter 12

Nurturing the Unborn Child

While the child is in the womb there is much that both father and mother can do to nurture the child and each other. This time of joyful anticipation should be used to its fullest potential. After all, you have a completely captive audience!

There is a story told in India about the great sage Shankaracharya who was such a highly evolved soul that not only was he fully conscious while in the womb, but while in there he taught the scriptures to his mother through intuitive communication. While this is certainly more than most of us can hope for it illustrates a very important point. The ability to communicate with the unborn child is a reality and not just an intriguing idea. It is a reality that is based on deep spiritual teachings. In fact, the growing child isn't just taking in nutrients through the umbilical cord but is soaking up the sounds, thoughts and experiences of the mother.

The ability to hear is one of the first senses to awaken in the infant. Along with physical hearing is the vibrational receptivity of the soul. Be careful about the type of music you listen to during this time. Just as I mentioned before, avoid loud, fast music. Try to listen to music that expresses the more refined qualities in life. Joyous harmonies and uplifting melodies, these are the music for the unborn. The same holds true for television and movies. Take in only wholesome entertainment.

Can you teach your child to speak a foreign language while in the womb? Probably not, but as a potential it does exist.

There are many amazing things in life that people are quick to scoff at because we haven't been able to prove them in the scientific laboratory. And to add to the hypocrisy of the so called "logic of the skeptical mind" there are many things that have been scientifically proven that people still don't want to believe!

Therese Neumann was a Christian mystic in Konnersreuth, Bavaria, in the last century. She was so closely attuned to Jesus Christ that in mystical union with Christ she received the stigmata - the wounds of Christ. As a result of this experience she became so directly linked to the source of life within that she no longer needed to eat or drink. She was tested and observed in hospitals for weeks on end. No one ever saw her eat or drink. She would swallow only a small communion wafer each day. She lived this way for over 40 years – and she wasn't even skinny!

So what does this have to do with us ordinary people? Just that we cut ourselves off from so much of our potential because we don't even try. Just making an effort in the spiritual life is a major step forward. So try to communicate with your unborn child. Be creative and have fun.

One of the things that is a time-honored practice in India is the reading of the scriptures to the unborn child. I did this when Bhavani was pregnant. Though the twins have never indicated that they heard me I like to think that some of their sweet nature is due to this. In any case, Bhavani and I were certainly uplifted by the experience. We spent many happy hours together, her head on my lap while I read. It seems to me, that alone makes it a worthwhile endeavor.

Anything that showers uplifting vibrations upon mother and child can do nothing but be helpful, whether the child can consciously perceive it or not. And this isn't limited to just spiritual activities. Anything that brings a wholesome sense of joy, laughter and general good feeling should be considered as beneficial to mother and child.

There are some things that should definitely be avoided at this time. Mothers can do much physical and spiritual harm to themselves and their child if they do not abstain from using all types of drugs unless specifically prescribed by a doctor. Alcohol is also another dangerous drug to unborn children. If mother usually smokes cigarettes it is strongly recommended that she abstain at this time. This isn't a bad idea for the father either. Maybe this can be the final reason to quit! Even the caffeine in many drinks should be avoided if possible.

Drugs and alcohol are not only physically dangerous but spiritually harmful. They pull the mind down and make us more sense bound rather than uplifted. The desire to use intoxicants is tied to the ego's urge to escape stress and loneliness. God's presence is the only lasting cure for these symptoms. The illusions of sensory pleasures will never satisfy the soul.

Along with the avoidance of anything that is generally agitating to the mind, try to avoid anger. Anger is a very powerful force for harm in this world. The sound of an angry voice isn't only unpleasant to the ears but hurtful to the soul. It upsets everyone; including the unborn child.

The spiritual root of anger is thwarted desires. No matter the age of the person, most expressed anger is like the temper tantrum of a child without self-control. Life doesn't go the way that we want it to go, so that makes us angry. Certainly

Positive Flow Childbirth

there are many ways that people arrive at anger and sometimes it can be personally healing or righteous. But those instances are much rarer than your regular run of the mill "I can't control myself" anger.

Just as we broadcast our loving invitation before conception, now that the child is in the womb it is easier to focus our energies on this particular soul. Continue sending your loving thoughts. Mother and father can even place their hands over the child inside. Feel your loving God-given energy flowing through your hands and to the child. Then take a moment to mentally rest in the oneness of Spirit.

Chapter 13

Energization

There are certain physical practices that you can start right away that will be of general benefit. Later on we will discuss how these efforts help provide a base from which to approach the labor itself.

Exercise should be regular and energetic – at least ½ hour each day as long as your physician doesn't prescribe against it. Many mothers have run marathons well into pregnancy. Walking, tennis, bike riding, you can do almost anything that you normally do to keep fit as long as you feel up to it. Just try to avoid sports where there is high impact or an excessive risk of injuring yourself. Swimming is particularly good because the water eases the effect of gravity.

Think of yourself as being in training. Even though your body will become larger and you will naturally be more protective of your body during this time, you need to do your best to be in good shape. There is a certain athletic reality to giving birth. You will need strength and stamina.

While exercising make special efforts to breathe deeply. Remember when we talked about the link between life and breath, how the breath is activated by cosmic energy coming in through the medulla at the base of the brain? Take time to become more aware of life's universal life force as it flows into your body through the medulla. Try to feel that this cosmic force rather than the food that you eat is animating your life.

The great Master of yoga, Paramhansa Yogananda, developed a series of Energization Exercises that are extremely helpful for learning to consciously feel and direct the cosmic energy into and through your body. They enable you to energize your body at will. Here are a couple of the exercises so that you can start consciously vitalizing your body and mind right away.

Double Breath

A double breath is a short and then long inhalation through the nose followed by a short and then long exhalation through the mouth. Breathe in through the nose, short/long, and then out through the mouth, short/long. When you practice this hold the breath for the count of three before you exhale. So you go in/innn through the nose, hold for the count of three and then exhale out/ouuut through the mouth. Repeat three times.

Whole Body Energization

This exercise is for recharging the whole body. Stand with your feet at shoulder width apart. Extend your arms forward at shoulder height so that your palms are touching. Then bend your knees slightly. Now inhale with a double breath. As you inhale gradually tense all of the muscles in the whole body simultaneously as you straighten the legs and spread your arms out to your sides. As you tense the muscles, do so in a flow: low, medium, high - hold at high tension for the count of three. Then exhale with a double breath and relax the muscles high, medium, low, relaxed.

When tensing your arms while they spread out to the sides also close and tense your fists. Once the whole body is tense, the legs are straight and the arms extended out to the sides, hold the breath and keep the tension at a high level for three counts, feeling all you your cells being energized and vitalized. Then exhale with a double breath through the mouth as you gradually relax the muscles back into your starting position.

While this a lot to think about at first, with practice it will become quite natural. Be sure to increase the tension from low, medium, to high, at a gradual pace. Then decrease the tension in reverse, from high, medium, low and then relax. When teaching this exercise Paramhansa Yogananda used to say, "Tense with will, relax and feel." He also said, "The greater the will, the greater the flow of energy." Practice recharging the whole body three to five times. You can do this as often as you like during the day.

You can also recharge the body while lying in bed before you get up in the morning. Do it just the same as described above, except don't move the arms or legs - tense and relax them in a comfortable position at your sides. Visualize the universal life force coming in through the medulla as you do the double breath and tense the whole body, low, medium, high, holding the breath for three counts once you have reached high tension. Then exhale with the double breath and relax from high, medium, low until fully relaxed. This is a great way to wake the body up!

This idea of consciously drawing on the inner life force is very important in the spiritual life. It is this life force that provides us with the energy to accomplish whatever we attempt in life. By learning to increase our awareness of it and consciously draw on it we will begin to access more and more of it. As you will see, this is going to be very helpful when it comes time for the very challenging task of giving birth to a child. Additionally, when we learn to turn this life force back

Positive Flow Childbirth

towards its source through meditation and right living we can dramatically speed up our journey towards self-realization.

Chapter 14

Relaxation

Along with energizing the body there is the need to withdraw energy from the body. Relaxation is necessary both physically and mentally so that we can help the process of birth rather than make it more difficult. While you are practicing the energization exercises, when you begin to relax the muscles feel that you are turning off the energy and withdrawing it back to the medulla.

This conscious turning off of the energy is just as important as the ability to turn it on. The tensions of daily life build up within us and strengthen the ripples of restlessness that keep our minds from reflecting pure Spirit. While it is true that some tensions come from the variety of ways that we use and/or abuse our bodies, the stresses in the mind also cause many of the tensions that we experience in the body. You know what I mean: Like that spot in your neck or back that hurts after you have had a hard day or an argument.

Retained mental stress can cause stomach ulcers and lead to heart disease. Even some forms of cancer can be caused or exacerbated by stress. In fact, many diseases gain a foothold in our bodies because our body's energy patterns are weakened by various types of stress and their corresponding tensions. It is interesting to note that the very word disease (dis-ease) speaks of its roots in this higher understanding.

Retained muscle tension can come from overexertion of the muscles, like the way you feel after using muscles you aren't used to using. But unless you have strained or injured a muscle that type of tension will go away with no lasting negative effect. The buildup of longstanding tensions in the body is harmful to mental, physical and spiritual well-being. The more tension we carry the more difficult it is to free our minds from excessive body consciousness, thus binding the soul more firmly to this bag of bones in which we currently reside.

There are a number of ways to help the release of these built-up tensions. All of the techniques that we have discussed so far will be a benefit in this area, so keep them in mind as we add some more.

Water

Water is a healing element in nature. It can be used in many ways, everything from drinking it to bathing in it. There are health spas all around the world that claim the healing powers of their waters. While it is unlikely that all of those claims are equally true, it is also unlikely that none of them are true.

Whether it be from a spa, swimming pool or bath tub we all have experienced how water can relax the body and mind. Seek opportunities to immerse your body in water. Along with lessening the effects of gravity the warm water provides an excellent environment for consciously releasing your tensions by mentally expanding them out of your body into the water.

Heat

Heat has also been used since time immemorial for the releasing of tension. A sauna or steam bath can be very beneficial. They help us to sweat out many impurities and tensions in the body. Heat can penetrate deeply into the muscles and tissues around the nerves which increases beneficial circulation of the blood. As you enjoy the heat, mentally feel that it is purifying not only your body, but that it is also cleansing your mind and spirit.

One thing you have to be somewhat careful about while pregnant is not changing your body temperature too drastically for an extended period of time. So take care when using therapies that can affect your body's core temperature. Common sense should be applied copiously. You don't want to cause tension by overdoing your efforts to minimize tension!

Massage

Another very pleasant way to release physical and mental stress is with a massage. There are many types of massage. I would caution you against massage that is so deep that it really hurts. A little discomfort in the muscles of some areas of the body is normal, but if the pressure makes you cry out in pain... consider asking the therapist to not press so hard. You should feel better afterwards because it felt good, not because you were glad it was over! Massage therapists who have been trained in understanding the energy flows of the body are much more effective than those who just give the old fashioned rub down type of massage. You might want to try a few different styles and therapists until you find the right fit for you.

During the massage try to consciously release the tensions. Don't leave it just to the massage therapist. Mentally go into the muscles and consciously release the tensions. This conscious participation can really help. One of the benefits of using your own awareness to consciously release the tensions is that you are working from the inside out rather than the outside in. Try to visualize the tension expanding out of your body.

Yoga Postures

Again I would like to mention the Yoga Postures (Asana).

Positive Flow Childbirth

This science is based on a deep knowledge of the energy flows that make up the body. Each posture is designed to massage not only the muscles from the *inside out* but to create energy patterns that help to balance the energies of the body and mind. The Yoga Postures also help to release harmful energies, be they mental, physical or spiritual. There are many good books and videos available. I particularly recommend *Ananda Yoga for Self Awareness* by Swami Kiryananda. I also encourage you to attend a class if possible. Not only will personalized instruction be helpful, but the group energy will give you added enthusiasm and support for your practice.

Bhavani had been practicing and teaching Hatha Yoga for about 15 years at this time. She continued leading her classes until the beginning of the ninth month. Of course she couldn't do all of the postures the same as before, but she made little adjustments and got excellent results.

Some people teach that you shouldn't invert the body during pregnancy and others teach that many of the poses need to be drastically modified. It is Bhavani's opinion, as well as my own, that as long as you use common sense and pay careful attention to how your body is responding, you should do a pose the way it is supposed to be done as long as it feels beneficial to you. If you need to make little adjustments fine, but it isn't necessary to create a whole new set of poses just because you are pregnant. It isn't that it is *wrong* to do so, it just isn't absolutely necessary to do so.

Something that many yoga teachers do not stress enough is the importance of relaxation during yoga practice. During each pose, and especially after each pose, try to inwardly withdraw and release the energy in the body just the way we talked about with massage. You should do this with the energization exercises as well. The principle is to consciously enter into the area of tension and release that energy consciously by mentally expanding it out of the body.

Deep Relaxation Technique

After you have done a set of yoga postures or anytime that you want to relax deeply you can practice this technique.

Lay down on your back with your arms comfortably at your sides palms upward.

Practice the full body recharging exercise that we learned in the last chapter. You will keep your arms at your sides while you do this. Inhale with a double breath while tensing the whole body, exhale with a double breath and relax. Do this two or three times.

Now make sure you are comfortable with arms at your sides and palms facing up.

We will now consciously withdraw the energy from the body. Just like flipping a light switch we will mentally turn off the energy in all of your muscles one area at a time. Start with the feet. Mentally relax them completely. Just mentally switch off the energy and release your mental attachment to your feet. Then do this same which each successive area: the calves, the thighs, the buttocks, the lower back and abdomen, the upper back and chest, the hands and forearms, the upper arms, the shoulders, the neck, and the head. Be sure that once you have switched off the energy in a body part you don't turn it on again by moving it. You must be absolutely still. It will take some practice.

Once the whole body is relaxed with the energy withdrawn try to feel peace vibrating all through your body like waves washing on the shore. Then expand this awareness of peace in all directions. Let it fill the room and reach down into the floor and out towards the walls and ceiling. Continue expanding while you mentally reach out beyond the building

Positive Flow Childbirth

and deep into the earth. Expand your peace up into the sky and gradually outward to fill the state, the country and the whole world. Then keep on going out into space until you fill the whole universe with your consciousness of infinite peace. Let yourself rest in this expanded awareness of peace for as long as you like.

When you feel to, slowly bring yourself back into the body. Don't jump up! Take some time to gently turn the energy back on in the muscles. Gently wiggle your toes and then rock your head side to side. When you feel to, sit up. Take a moment while you are sitting to meditate for a few minutes. Remember that expanded awareness of peace and let your heart expand in that same way. The infinite consciousness of love, peace and joy is your true higher Self. Make friends with this universal Self and it will change your life in ways that you never would have imagined.

Now try to carry this inner peace into the rest of your day. Let all of your thoughts and actions reflect little glimmers of that universal peace. And of course, remember there is a little one inside you sharing it with you!

Chapter 15

Natural or UnNatural Childbirth?

Before we discuss the medical and birthing options that you will have to decide upon it is essential that we review the basis from which we can evaluate our decisions. The most reliable and firm foundation for making choices in life is self-honesty. It isn't enough to look at life idealistically with a view of the way we want things to be and then just push forward blindly without a thought for anything else. Desire alone cannot manifest our dreams. We need to apply the God-given attributes of intelligence and common sense along with intuitive perception.

I used to think that the ultimate image of birth was of the Native American Indian women who would go out into the forest and quietly give birth on their own. No muss or fuss, just an incredibly strong and controlled woman meeting nature's way head on. I don't really know if my mental image was common or unusual. The history of what has taken place before our times tends to be very unreliable. But I am sure of one thing; the infant and/or mother mortality rate was much higher at that time.

So does this mean that we just submit to the ways of Western medicine in the name of what is commonly done today?

Positive Flow Childbirth

Absolutely not! It simply means that we need to throw out our fantasies about the way we think things should be and carefully evaluate each aspect of the process with the best balance of inner and outer understanding that we can muster.

Many people have somehow gotten the impression that Western medicine is by its nature unnatural. Is it unnatural to use silverware? Is it unnatural to use tools? Are blenders, telephones and automobiles unnatural? They are all made of elements found in nature to which God-given human intelligence and will has been applied.

What does natural really mean? Most people would say that natural is that which is found in nature unchanged. Yet what is found in nature? Things that change all of the time! Life itself is by its own nature change. That is the one thing that we can always count on in this physical world: Things will change.

If a sea otter uses a rock to open its abalone dinner that is natural. But if mankind uses a can opener that is not natural? This is where we again need to leave the "It must be exactly this or that!" way of thinking. How can any part of life be less than a part of life? There is no way to say that mankind's evolution is not a part of nature. All life on this planet must by definition be a part of nature.

The real question is whether or not we are expressing the underlying positive energies of life that flow towards a higher more harmonious understanding of life as Spirit or expressing a more limited selfish ego-promoting fear based disharmonious flow away from Spirit.

It isn't always easy to evaluate any given situation in this light because many of life's challenges are a mixture of expanding and contracting energies. In most situations we will need to look at the sum total of the end result and see what it gives us. The only caveat to this is that we must understand that the end doesn't always justify the means. The solution to hunger in the world can never be to kill people. Certainly fewer people would help the situation but can killing people in the name of ending hunger possibly be a right action? No.

Actions that are based in truth are always beneficial. That doesn't mean that they are always easy or that they never involve suffering. But they always express the highest understanding of truth that we are able to see at that time.

Every person travels a different path through life so we each need to be able to perceive truth individually as it applies to the unique circumstances of our lives. That which is a right decision for one person may not be the correct decision for another. As an example. It would be generally agreed that it is an act of unselfish sacrifice to give up one's life to save another's. But there are circumstances that can come up in life where the sacrifice is to live and not to die. Imagine the survivors of a shipwreck. If one sailor adrift on the ocean in a small lifeboat with others who do not know the ways of the sea stops eating first and dies, all may perish. But if the sailor stays alert and continues to do those things that may help then all or some may be saved. This is not an easy choice.

That is why we should be careful not to let past preconceived images of that which is right distort our evaluation of current circumstances. Set the highest course you can and then flow with it. Changes may need to be made midstream. Don't let your desire for the way you would prefer things to be, keep you from staying in the most positive flow that you can. Remember, your right attitude and efforts of attunement to higher consciousness are every bit as important as the individual decisions themselves.

The key to making the best possible decisions in our lives is to have developed some real inner-communication links with our Creator. So many people wait until disaster is at their door to turn towards God. Develop an inner relationship with your very best Divine Friend who happens to be the source of infinite wisdom and love. Don't wait until things are too tough to handle on your own to turn towards God - although it is also true that any time is a good time to turn towards God. The best of times are all the sweeter when we can share them with our best friends. And there is no friend closer or truer than our friend, beloved God.

Chapter 16

Conscious or UnConscious Labor?

The way that mothers experience bringing a child into this world can differ quite dramatically. One extreme is that of the mother totally sedated in an antiseptic delivery room while people she has never seen before help her with the delivery. She wakes up hours after the birth to be informed as to how things went. Another example is the mother who has the baby in some unexpected place like a cab with no trained medical supervision. Some mothers don't have any help at any time during their pregnancy while others are supported extensively from day one.

A question that comes to mind is: Did these mothers choose those conditions? Or were they just riding the wave of life as it flows by and passively hoping for the best?

When Bhavani had two children years before I met her she was like the first story. At the time she didn't realize that she could actually make choices about the way things were handled. She was wheeled into the delivery room and upon crossing that threshold she relinquished all control of the situation. She was never consulted. She was shaved, sedated and told the results when she woke up. Not a very dignified way to be treated.

Fortunately the human body and spirit is able to withstand the many insults that we receive in life. Those two children have grown up to be fine healthy individuals. But by the time this new pregnancy came along Bhavani had learned much about the alternatives and chose to have a totally different experience. This is a key point: Making a conscious choice. Looking at the options and saying: That's the one for me. Being aware of what is going on in life is essentially important to the expansion of our consciousness. When people live out of touch with life they lose their ability to make choices.

Can you believe that some women have had babies without even knowing that they were pregnant? It is true. I heard the story of a woman who was just lying in her bed and thought that she was passing gas. When she noticed it was wet down there she looked and found a baby! I don't mean to put her down but it is essential that we be awake and ready in life if we want to get the most out of it. That woman was seriously disconnected from what was going on in her life.

There are times in life when we will have to surrender to circumstances, but even then we should consciously make the choice to surrender. Don't let life take control of you! Be the master of your own destiny by acting with Divinely-guided conscious will. Take the time to consider all of your birthing options before you make a decision. Then be prepared to make adjustments as things develop.

One of the goals of the spiritual life is to be always even-minded and cheerful. Take this attitude into your birthing experience. Try to make your decisions without fretting. If things get difficult or don't go the way you expected keep your good cheer. This positive way of reacting to challenges is one of the differences between those who live successfully and those who just live.

As we look at some of your options keep in mind that the right choices for you may be different than those that are right for someone else. There isn't just one right way to do it. Think about how you can blend the different possibilities in a way that resonates with your own inner sense of rightness.

Sometimes we think that God doesn't want us to have things our way, that we are supposed to suffer for spiritual growth. The fulfillment of wholesome desires is not against the principles of truth. It is only our attachment to having or not having them the way we would prefer that gets us into trouble. So, as you try to make things the best that you can, also stay a little detached. That way if things change - which they most often do - you won't be overly upset by it.

One of the exciting things about living in today's times is that there are so many choices. The advances in medicine, transportation and communication have made it possible to do things now that weren't even thought of not all that many years ago. So as you explore the possibilities keep an open mind and have fun visualizing yourself in a variety of situations until you find one that feels just right for you.

Chapter 17

Western Medicine: Sin or Savior?

For many on the spiritual path there is confusion as to how Western medicine fits into a spiritual and/or wholistic approach to life. Let's take some time to look at this in relation to our decisions about health in general and childbirth in particular.

In order to understand the healing process in the body we need to remember that the energies inside the body are what activate the body's ability to respond to the environment in which we live. It is the application of energy to anything in life that allows change to occur. Positive energy results in positive change, and likewise, negative energies bring about negative change.

The physical harm that comes to the body operates just on the surface of who we are. Underneath that physical harm is still an energy pattern. It is the balance between the severity of the injury and the strength of our energy pattern that will determine how serious the problem will be. Ultimately, as spiritual beings we have the capability to heal ourselves instantly through the application of positive will. Though as a practical matter, few people have attained personal mastery of this potential.

The reality of the underlying energy pattern in the body can be seen with people who have lost limbs. They often claim that they can still feel the limb even though it isn't there. Researchers chalk this up to some kind of nerve reaction. The fact is that the energy pattern of the lost limb is still there and it is through this energy pattern that the awareness of the limb continues.

How do lizards regenerate their tails? There are other animals that regenerate body parts as well. And how is it that the human body grows into the shape that it does in the first place? Is it just chromosomes?

The central truth is that the physical body follows the patterns of thought and energy carried in the causal and astral bodies. These subtle bodies energize the physical body and determine its shape. If, through the application of will, we activate the "grow a limb energy", then a lost limb can actually be grown back. But needless to say, this ability is not an easy one to achieve or many would avail themselves of it.

When our bodies fight off an infection we generally aren't immediately conscious of the battle going on inside. The body seems to get going on its own. That is done through unconscious will. We only perceive the symptoms, such as a swollen and reddened body part or a fever after the microscopic battle has been engaged. It is important to understand that it is the stimulation of the energy flow through either conscious or unconscious will that actually activates and supports the healing process in the body.

What can we do to help ourselves since we haven't yet learned to tap the full potential of our inner resources? As always, we can turn to God. The acknowledgement of this inner relationship will align us with the positive flow of energy that God is always sending to us. Also, remember that God has created this world as an expression of His infinite consciousness and the efforts of mankind to understand the body from the outside are also part of this Divine drama.

What physicians have discovered from time immemorial is that there are physical things that can be done to stimulate and guide the healing process. But, unfortunately, many physicians see the physical process only and do not align that physical understanding with a deeper spiritual/wholistic understanding.

In the East, medicine over the centuries has concentrated on the inner energy flows of the body. In India there is the science of Ayurveda and in China there are numerous healing modalities that have been passed down through the centuries. The unifying feature of all these Eastern approaches to healing is that they start with understanding inner energy flows and then work in a variety of mental, physical and spiritual ways to stimulate positive energetic changes in the body, mind and spirit. The goal is to align the patients consciousness/energy patterns with the divine healing power.

In the West, medicine has concentrated on the physical aspects of the body and the advances that Western medicine has accomplished should not be discounted just because they don't include the whole picture. When my sister was in labor with her son it was found that the baby's head had grown too large for the pelvis: a vaginal exit was not going to happen. By performing a Cesarean section operation both mother and child were spared certain death. There is nothing unspiritual about that.

If you get in a serious car accident Western medicine has the practical skills to get you going again. We need to give credit where credit is due.

The problem arises from the tendency of Western medicine to poke its head into places where it isn't needed or to dismiss a wide variety of wholistic approaches to healing without any scientific support for their disdain. Separate from the unfortunate fact that many hospitals and physicians do unnecessary procedures to help their financial bottom line and disguise this practice in the name of being thorough, is the lack of training by Western physicians in the Eastern approach to healing. Certainly there has been progress in this area and there is a growing number of physicians that are trained in both Eastern and Western medicine.

The truth is that neither Eastern nor Western approaches have perfect records in either outcomes or ethics. Each circumstance must be weighed in the moment in order to understand the best total approach to any given situation. And it is ultimately the recipient of health care that must determine which path to follow.

Another factor that isn't often enough considered is that by constantly stimulating the body from the outside we lessen our ability to use our inner resources. We begin to think that the medicine is what makes us well. We begin to affirm: I am a body and things outside myself are necessary for healing. This is the real harm that comes from overuse of any kind of medicinal aids. Using our God-given abilities to their utmost is essential for developing the strength of energy flow and will power that it takes to achieve true self-realization.

So use medical help as needed but don't let it intrude on your ability to tap your own inner resources. Only the necessary level of intervention should be seen as the criteria with which you evaluate your decisions. Use your best judgment taking into account all of the medical options that you are presented. Don't relinquish your right to decide unless you are incapacitated.

What can easily happen to mothers is that in the intensity of the moment they lose control of the situation.

Positive Flow Childbirth

Having your mate there to be your voice on issues that you have discussed ahead of time is very helpful. And making sure that the medical staff knows your basic wishes before things get started is essential. You may want to consider creating a Living Will that spells out your medical wishes in case there isn't a legally acceptable person on site to make medical decisions for you.

Some mothers have had the birth of their child prematurely induced just because the doctor was in a hurry! Make sure that you feel comfortable with what is going on. Don't let procedures take place without you and/or your coach being advised as to what is happening. This is part of your commitment to being conscious during the experience. It also points out the need to choose the right medical help. They should be people who are easy to communicate with and who you feel you can trust.

Physical intervention when the body and mind are not capable of overcoming the potential harmful effects of a situation is a great blessing, one that comes from man's attunement to the knowledge of the universe. Think of the countless benefits Western medicine has brought to mankind. The advances of Western medicine manifest the positive moving forward of mankind's evolution. But it must be understood that as long as the soul is unaware of its nature as Spirit, then even if science gave each person a thousand years to live true happiness would not be found.

Finding the balance between doing it on your own and utilizing medical support is not a simple equation. But with much research, discussion and inner attunement, a picture of what is right for you will begin to develop.

No matter what you decide, after you have utilized your very best efforts in trying to understand and follow your highest truth, give the results to God. Whatever happens, rest in the knowledge that God's view of our lives is much larger than our own. We can't see all of the combinations of energies from the past that bring us to any given experience in the present. Remember, every experience in life is a step closer to union with the Divine if we take it in the right spirit. Let your acceptance of God's will in your life be the overriding view from which you see everything.

God is the giver of all things. Let us rest in the wisdom of His choice of gifts for us.

Chapter 18

Prenatal Care

There is one course of action that has shown itself to be of consistent value to all expectant mothers and that is good prenatal care. Once you know you are pregnant do not delay in getting connected with qualified medical support professionals whose experience can help you very much. Actually, this is something that should also be considered in the very beginning of your decision to have a child. Do you live in an area where you can get the level of support that you would prefer?

Some people may decide to do things on their own, especially if they live in a very rural area. It should be taken into account that there is a risk of problems during childbirth. Many of those problems are not in the least bit life threatening to mother or child when experienced help is available. Without that help small problems may escalate, to say nothing of problems that can be big from the start.

There are a wide variety of books available on the physical aspects of childbirth and much study and reflection should be done before the decision is made to do things completely on your own. For those who do plan on using professional help – I say professional because just having your mate or friend nearby who has been to a few births isn't the same as having someone who has made a study of the subject and has practical experience – it is important to get connected with such a person as soon as possible. Don't forget to make sure that the people who you are planning on having at the birth will be available when you need them.

When looking for a medical support team it is important to keep in mind the principles of harmony that we have talked about earlier. While discussing things maintain an inner connection to your higher Self and ask: How does this feel? As you shop for help – and you should shop – you might want to make a list of things that are important to you. This list should include physical, educational and vibrational concerns.

When choosing medical help ascertain what facilities and/or resources do the candidates have at their disposal? What else can they draw on as needed? What do their services include? How many prenatal visits are included and how much time will they spend with you during each visit? What if they are sick or helping someone else when you need them? Who will cover?

What are their fees and are there any other possible expenses? What educational materials or programs do they offer? What is their basic philosophy towards medical issues having to do with childbirth? What decisions will they allow you to make before and during the birth? What is their educational background and their experience? Will they provide you with references? You can also check with the American Medical Association if you want to do so. Take the time before you go into a candidates office and consider this list. Add to this list any other areas of concern that come to mind.

The amount of time that this person is going to spend with you is very important. It indicates in many ways the quality of the care that you will be receiving. While it doesn't in itself indicate a person's technical ability it does say something about their character. This is a person who may have to make life and death decisions concerning you and your child. You want to make sure that you trust him/her. One of the strongest recommendations that you can get is from a friend who has had a child. Find out who they used and if they were satisfied with the care they received.

After you have done your research and checked out all of the possibilities take some time to let the information settle. Try to remember what it was like being in the doctor's or midwife's office. How did you feel there? Was it inviting, comforting and supportive? Or was it clinical and uncaring? Did you wait a really long time? Did you ask how many other mothers are they working with that will be due around the same time as you? Sometimes too busy is just as bad as not busy enough. Then with some detachment try and feel inside your self if one or another sticks out in your mind as the one that feels the best.

This sense of harmonious feeling is something that takes some time to develop. It shouldn't just be the reaction to a pleasant personality. Try to feel it as a deeper sense of correctness. Look for a feeling that resonates with an inner calmness in your heart.

Let God be a part of your decision. Pray about it. Ask for a sign. And then be watchful for the answer. For if you pray with concentration and sincerity an answer will surely come.

Chapter 19

Doctor or Midwife? Home or Hospital?

There are a number of factors that should be considered when trying to decide whether to use a doctor or midwife. Given that a totally natural birth will be our baseline goal, we must look at what level of support we will need to achieve as close to this result as we can. For some mothers, known medical conditions will make a vaginal birth impossible. The acceptance of this reality should not lessen your desire to make every other aspect of the experience as vibrationally high as possible. Rather than thinking of what can't be done, concentrate on what can be done.

The use of a physician and the best medical support team available should always be seen as the right action when faced with known impediments to the possibility of a medically unassisted birth. There is nothing unspiritual about protecting the life of the mother and child. Unnecessary risks should be seen as presuming on rather than having faith in God's protection.

On the other hand, we shouldn't live in fear. Many people choose hospital births just because they are afraid of things going wrong. Or because hospitals and doctors in the name of self-interest may exaggerate the dangers of something going wrong. If you have paid close attention to how the pregnancy is progressing and the medical advice that you have received says that everything is fine, there is no reason to fear having a child away from the hospital unless there is a specific contraindication. That doesn't mean that you don't plan for emergencies! It just means that we shouldn't live our lives in fear.

So assuming that your medical needs or the availability of other options don't limit your choices let's look at some of the possibilities. Deciding where you want to have the birth will have an effect on who you can get to help. Since we are basing our discussion on minimizing intervention let's start with a home birth and then work towards a hospital birth.

Many physicians today will not do home deliveries. So if you want a physician to help at home you will have to find one that is willing, otherwise you will have to find a midwife.

It is important to understand that not all midwives have the same level of training and experience. Some have had formal training and have been evaluated by a medically recognized organization. Others may have learned through experience by attending births. I'm not saying that one is automatically better than the other. I am saying check into it. Find out what qualifications the midwife has and use that information as part of your evaluation process.

The best time to deal with potential problems is before they happen. Does that sound familiar? So consider how much time this person is going to take to evaluate how you are doing. It isn't just a question of catching medical problems. It is also the psychological support that comes from really getting to know this person and not just being a number at the counter. This personal touch is very much a part of keeping the vibrations high.

Doctor or Midwife? Home or Hospital?

The back up support network that the midwife has is also very important. When our twins were born we actually had three midwives in attendance; one each for Bhavani and the two babies. This kind of planning ahead is essential if you want to have a home birth.

Making sure that the midwife has already thought of every possibility will give you more confidence that she knows what she is doing. Asking about logistical kinds of issues will give a feel for how she thinks and what her resources are. What physician will be called in if there is a problem? Or will it be the attending physician at the local emergency room who will help?

Discuss the type of birthing environment that you want to have and make sure that the midwife feels comfortable with your plans. There is a wide variety in the way people approach childbirth. Some make a party of it with music and lots of friends. Others want to have the baby underwater. Some want to wear clothes and others do not. Think about what you want. Read a book that specializes in discussing birthing options. Evaluate the different options in the light of your personal interests and preferences along with their compatibility with the uplifting vibrations that we have been talking about.

Some licensed midwives actually have hospital privileges and if the need arises can go with you to the hospital and assist the physician. In other cases the midwife can use a delivery room in the hospital and the doctor only attends if there is a problem. This can be a good alternative for those who like things as homey as possible but want or need the close support of medical facilities.

There are quite a few hospitals now that have what they call home birthing rooms where it is decorated like a bedroom: music, video, everything you could ask for. But keep in mind the vibrations that underlie the physical space. Is it calm? Is it

Positive Flow Childbirth

peaceful? Could you make it so with the right touches? Who will be allowed to attend with you?

Each doctor will have their own standards as to what they feel comfortable with. And many hospitals have rules that the doctors must follow. Find out ahead of time exactly what procedures will be followed under as many different types of situations as you can think of. If the doctor doesn't want to take the time to discuss these issues with you then take that into account as you decide with whom you want to work.

Remember, there isn't only one right way to do this. Let your instincts guide your search for the right situation. Don't give up on you ideal until you have exhausted every possibility. Here again, honesty is the best policy. So you think that a home birth is best but you can't quite face the challenges? Don't kid yourself. Take into account the harsh cold facts. Add to that your best inner feelings as to what is the right thing to do. Then stir it all up with lots of prayer.

You will find that the right solution to any question is at your disposal if you consult the source of all wisdom - the positive flow of Spirit. As a part of God all knowledge is available to you, all you need to do is practice tuning in to it.

Once you have set your course; be strong. Believe in the choices that you have made. That doesn't mean don't be open to change. It means that if you can feel the strength of the universe flowing through you there is a good chance that you are on the right track. Walk forward with humble confidence, while always listening for His voice.

Chapter 20
Life/Breath/Energy

It is interesting that in India there is one word for life, breath and energy: prana. Looking at the reason for this will help us understand more about how to prepare for labor. As we discussed earlier, it is the cosmic energy flowing into the body through the medulla that animates our lives. As this prana flows up and down the subtle inner spine it causes the physical breath to respond. When the energy flows up the spine we inhale. When the energy flows down the spine we exhale. Under most circumstances, when this energy ceases to flow the breath stops in the body and we say that physical life has ended.

There is a subtle link between the mind and the breath that is very important for spiritual growth. This connection will also give us a clue as to what we can do to help during labor. Have you ever noticed that when your mind is agitated you breathe more quickly? How about when you are angry? Emotions of passion have always been associated with the panting of the breath. Conversely, have you ever noticed that when your mind is very focused the breath is calm? Think about doing a very delicate task like threading a needle or building a ship in a bottle. You can't do it if your breath isn't calm. As you concentrate on the task the focusing of the mind calms the breath.

Positive Flow Childbirth

We talked earlier about how when the mind is calm it can reflect perfectly the consciousness of Spirit. But when we are not calm then the ripples of our restlessness keep us from the inner perceptions for which our souls long. When the mind becomes calm our energy withdraws from the senses into the inner spine. This turning of the awareness from outside the body to our inner awareness is what we are accomplishing as we practice meditation.

In order to speed up the process of interiorization we can learn to take control of the energy as it enters the body and direct it with the application of will power as we choose. We practiced one example of this when we discussed the energization exercises. In those exercises we are using the energy to recharge the physical body. There is another kind of exercise that does the same thing for the inner spine. It is called pranayama. Prana means life/breath/energy and yama means control. So when we practice pranayama we are consciously controlling the life energy within us through our connection to the breath.

Some people have translated the meaning of pranayama as breathing exercises but this is a limited view of what it really means. Yes, breathing exercises are involved. But if it is left just at that than a vast reservoir of understanding and capability is left behind. The breath is used to awaken and connect our awareness of this inner energy as it flows through the physical body and the subtle astral body. If we just do breathing exercises without the awareness of the subtle inner energy flow we will never make the transfer to perceiving the energy as the activating force. We will instead stay limited to the body and think that the breath is just a mechanism for delivering oxygen to the blood and expelling carbon dioxide.

By learning to control and harmonize ourselves with

this inner flow of energy we can do several very helpful things. The first is that we will be able to consciously calm our minds and begin to feel the natural peace of the soul. This alone is worth the effort. The next benefit is that as the mind calms so does the body. As our awareness is withdrawn into the inner spine the body relaxes, just like in the deep relaxation exercise that we practiced earlier. This combination of relaxation of the body and withdrawal of the mind from the senses to immerse itself in the peace of the soul is not only useful for Divine perceptions but also for childbirth.

Think about it. As the contractions start they aren't too bad. But as the process deepens it can be quite intense. Mental messages of rejection are sent out from the brain and the body often responds. Some women actually succeed in stopping the contractions for varying lengths of time because of the power of their mental resistance to what they are feeling. What the mother really needs to do is to relax instead of being tense. The idea is to flow *with* what the body is trying to do instead of resisting it.

But you say: It hurts!

Remember when we talked about transmuting sensual energy? We talked about drawing the sensations into and up the spine towards the brain so we can use it for spiritual growth instead of dissipating it through the senses. Well, that is just what needs to happen with the discomfort of the contractions. The mother should use the energy (sensations) of the contractions to increase her interiorization - mental withdrawal from sense awareness - so that not only does she disassociate herself from the pain but she increases the good positive energy flow in the spine; which helps all aspects of the process.

While withdrawing the energy into the spine the mother's consciousness should be turned towards God. What

Positive Flow Childbirth

greater source of comfort can we connect ourselves to during times of need? What happens is that the intensity of the birthing process is turned towards God communion. When successful, the result is a deeply comforting and calming experience instead of mental identification with intense physical pain.

Later on it will be time to come back into the body and consciously help with pushing the baby out. In the beginning stages, letting nature take its course and withdrawing into the spine is the way to go. The reason this works is because it is based on the way God created us. For every challenge in life there is a solution. When we actively align ourselves with the laws of the universe we will find many opportunities to turn potential discomfort toward peacefulness. For the process of birthing a child there can be no better course of action than using the very principles that have made and sustain our lives.

Chapter 21

Meditation
for Childbirth

In order to develop the necessary control over the breath and mind, efforts will need to begin much in advance of the birth. You can't expect to master these techniques in a few days or weeks. These techniques are not designed specifically for childbirth, they are basic to the way energy naturally flows in the body and can (should) be used as a regular part of one's spiritual practice. By recognizing that it is through the breath that we are held in the physical body we can begin through conscious effort to go beneath the surface of our physical existence and perceive more subtle realities.

Along with the techniques that I am sharing with you I recommend that you also explore using a breathing technique like the Bradley Method or Lamaze, which have both been used successfully. These different techniques don't have to be seen as competing with what we are discussing but should be seen as providing more options. You won't know until you get right down to trying exactly how things are going to go. Almost any proven technique can work if you apply yourself fully. The key will be: If you apply yourself!

As a practical matter, you may not have time to develop your use of all of the techniques that I am sharing with you.

Positive Flow Childbirth

It depends on when you are expecting and how deeply and regularly you apply yourself to the techniques.

With any breathing techniques that you use it is important to remember that if you have not prepared yourself through regular practice you run the risk of hyperventilating. Along with the danger of fainting is the associated spaciness of the mind. This loss of ability to concentrate and stay in control of your energies can be detrimental to the process. So remember what I said earlier, you will be in training. You need to take your efforts to be fully prepared seriously. It goes against our spiritual responsibility to do anything less than our very best. It's only then that we can rightfully turn to God in our times of need.

These techniques are so physically simple that you should beware of thinking: Oh, that's easy, no sweat! Remember, it is the awareness, the control of the inner energy and the focusing of the mind that we are after - not just the moving of air in the lungs. This is a very brief description of the technique. I encourage you to read my book Meditation: The Science and Art of Stillness for a more complete discussion of meditation.

Hong-Sau Meditation Technique

This technique is for calming the body and mind while becoming consciously connected to the energy flow in the spine. It is a technique for developing inner concentration that has been found effective for thousands of years in India. In this technique we DO NOT control the breath or the energy as it flows in the body. We "just watch it" with the complete attention of our awareness and attune ourselves to the flow of the breath.

Step 1 - Sit and Energize

To prepare for practicing the technique, sit up straight in a chair or sit on the floor. If you are on the floor, or even on some chairs, you may want to use a small cushion under the base of the spine for support. Do not lean back against anything. The spine should be as straight as possible. The hands should be relaxed palms upward on the thighs, the chin parallel to the floor and the shoulders pulled back slightly to keep the upper spine straight.

Begin by recharging the body with energy as we discussed in Chapter Thirteen. Inhale with a double breath, tense and energize the body, exhale and relax. Do this two or three times. Then consciously relax the body.

Step 2 - Equal Breathing

Now take a slow deep breath in through the nose counting to 6. Hold for 6 counts. Then exhale through the nose for 6 counts. Do this 3 times to begin with. As you feel comfortable with practice work up to 6 times. Make sure that the inhalation, hold and exhalation are all the same length of time. As you develop you ability then longer breaths are better. In the beginning 6-6-6 is fine but gradually as you can work up to 12-12-12 or even longer. If you become light headed it means you are overdoing it for the current state of your body. In that case, stop for now and next time do shorter segments and fewer repetitions.

Step 3 - Meditation

Now we are ready to begin our practice of the actual technique. After you have completed your last exhalation of the equal breathing give up control of the breath and let it proceed on its own. Do not control it. When it comes in by itself; let it. When it goes out by itself; let it. Do not in any way control it.

While the breath is moving in and out of its own accord there are two things that we want to do. The first is to consciously link the body and the mind. In order to do this we use a phrase or mantra. There are a number of ways you can do this, the important thing to remember is that you only say the words mentally and not out loud.

In India, they say Hong with the inhalation and Sau with the exhalation. The repeating of Hong Sau (I am He) is an affirmation of our oneness with infinite Spirit. It is better if you use the Sanskrit words Hong (the ong like song) Sau (sounds like saw) because these sounds are vibrationally attuned to the energy behind the breath as it flows in the spine, but you can experiment with the English (I am, with the inhalation, and He, with the exhalation) if you prefer.

You could also mentally say: I am peace or I am love. Any similar phrase will work. Christians can use: I love you, Jesus. Whatever you choose to use, remember, don't say it out loud. Say it mentally and stay with it. Don't let your mind wander. If you find that you have mentally wandered then gently bring your mind back to the mantra. If the breath pauses at either end then just relax and wait until it flows again of its own accord.

In the beginning you should watch the breath in the lungs but as you become more comfortable with the technique experiment with watching the breath where it enters and leaves the nasal cavity at the top of the nose. By watching it there you can also be aware of the energy at the spiritual eye (a point between and just slightly above the eyebrows).

The next step is to become aware of the subtle energy currents in the spine. When the breath comes in there is a rising of energy in the spine. And when the breath goes out the energy goes down the spine. It takes time to perceive this. Don't force it. Just relax and try to be receptive to perceiving the energy.

Concentration on the mantra that you are using, connected to the uncontrolled breath, should be your main focus. As you relax and deepen your practice over time you will begin to feel the inner energy flow and begin to identify it.

This technique not only develops one's concentration and awareness of inner peace, but it is so effective for expanding one's consciousness that many people have had great spiritual experiences through the deep practice of this technique.

This technique should normally be practiced with eyes closed. That doesn't mean you can't do it with eyes open sometimes, but for regular practice your eyes should be closed. Practice this technique morning and evening for at least five or ten minutes. Work your way up to fifteen or twenty minutes at each session. Even longer would be good. Add a session at noon if you can or a few minutes at any time during the day.

Step 4 - Sitting in the Silence

After practicing the technique sit in the silence and enjoy your awareness of inner peace. Sitting in the silence is a very important part of the technique. As our experience of inner stillness deepens we will begin to become more intuitively sensitive. This is the portal to inner communion with God. This technique will not only help in your preparations for giving birth, but it can transform your relationship with God. As you practice add your hearts devotion. Let each session be a humble offering of your desire to be ever more in tune with the Divine, until your affirmations of "I am He" become the realization that we are in truth: Spirit.

Chapter 22

Energy Control for Childbirth

Now that we have learned a technique of meditation/concentration we can begin to turn the focusing of the mind to actually controlling the energy. To do this we return to the principles of pranayama. Now we will actually control the energy as it comes into the body by taking control of the breath. Before we start the technique remember what the goal of our practice will be. We want to withdraw our awareness from the senses and escape for a time into the inner world of Spirit. This is not subconsciousness as in when we sleep. It is just the opposite: It is superconsciousness.

What is the difference between this technique and other breathing techniques that are used for childbirth? Most other techniques use the breath strictly as a focal point for pain management. The awareness stays in the body the whole time. While there is nothing wrong with that, it isn't as effective nor as vibrationally uplifting as inner withdrawal from the senses and connecting to a higher state of consciousness. By focusing your awareness in the inner spine, along with divorcing yourself from the identification with the discomfort you are consciously connecting into the source of the positive flow of life. This is a source of joy and inspiration that can lift you high above the difficulties of any of life's challenges: including the pain of childbirth.

Another alternative to explore is the use of hypnotherapy or self-hypnosis. This process is used to attain a state of inner withdrawal through guided visualization. It can be effective for those who don't have the time or inclination to apply themselves through the practice of pranayama.

To give you a realistic view of what I am trying to share with you I must mention that the exclusive use of these meditation techniques for childbirth isn't easy. Some women won't be able to rely on these techniques exclusively. It is dependent on how deep you as an individual are able to go into the technique.

These techniques represent a way that we can expand our inner horizons regardless of whether we can individually utilize them for all stages of the birthing process. Their practice leads to an experience of inner peace, calmness and clarity of mind. That is why I recommend using them, if necessary, in conjunction with more outward forms of breathing techniques for the birth. If you can use them exclusively as I'll describe the way Bhavani did: great! If you can't, then they will help you be more effective with whatever else you use.

The thing to remember is that if we don't know what the possibilities are we can't decide if they are for us or not. These techniques do work. Will they work for you? It depends on how successful you are at applying them. Explore the possibilities for yourself and then make a decision.

There is one other thing that I must mention to you before sharing this technique. Like many things that we do in life, when we are a beginner the technique that we use is slightly different than when we are advanced. The way that I am describing this technique is for beginners. It is not appropriate to share the advanced version of this technique without substantially more preparation and understanding on the part of the student. Additionally, I encourage students of these techniques to seek direct person to person instruction from a qualified instructor. Group practice of these techniques is also extremely beneficial.

The most effective technique that I am aware of for interiorizing one's consciousness is the technique of Kriya Yoga that was brought to America from India in 1920 by Paramhansa Yogananda - author of the spiritual classic *Autobiography of a Yogi*. Kriya Yoga is the technique of pranayama that Bhavani used for the birth of the twins. If you are interested in finding out more about the technique of Kriya Yoga please contact me through the publisher.

Before you practice this technique, prepare by practicing the Hong-Sau Technique for five or ten minutes. Once you are calm and interiorized you can begin your practice of Pranayama.

Pranayama for Childbirth

The foundation of this technique is the same as the equal breathing that we discussed in the last chapter. We will be controlling the breath in the same basic way but with a few differences. In this technique we inhale and exhale only through the mouth. Additionally, we only hold the breath for the count of 3.

To practice this technique start with the breath out. Just exhale and relax for a short moment before you begin. Slowly inhale through the mouth, hold the breath for 3 counts, and then exhale through the mouth. Don't forget that the inhalation and the exhalation should be of equal length. So you can start with 6-3-6 and work your way up to 12-3-12. Remember, we want to make the inhalation and exhalation as long as we can, but we don't want to get out of breath or lightheaded. If you get out of breath: Shorten the length of your breaths. If you get light headed: Discontinue your practice until it passes.

Lightheadedness is generally due to over oxygenation of the blood. Try doing just three to five repetitions of the technique numerous times during the day. Gradually your body will get used to this. If lightheadedness persists, check with your physician.

If this seems too easy don't worry, it will get harder as we discuss the deeper aspects of our efforts.

Now that you know what the lungs are doing, let's talk about the mouth. By restricting the air flow through the lips we are going to supercharge our efforts. What we need to do is restrict the air flow as it passes by the lips so that it helps us to create a slow and steady inhalation and exhalation. Keep in mind that while we do this we don't want any tension in the mouth or lips. Here are some ideas on how to do this. Do some experimentation until it becomes comfortable for you.

Let's start with some tension so that you can get a feel for the air flow first. Purse your lips like you were going to kiss someone. Then as you inhale and exhale adjust the size of the opening so that you get a smooth steady flow of air. This will give you a kind of hissing sound as you inhale and exhale.

The only problem with this way of doing it is that the lips are tense and that makes us more aware of the body and will be tiring over time. Try relaxing the lips and yet still keeping control of the air flow by adjusting the size of the opening of the lips. Make sure that the stream of air is slow and steady.

Another way to do it is to use your teeth as the point of constriction rather than your lips. Put your tongue right up against the front teeth of your lower jaw. With your lips relaxed and teeth not quite closed, draw the air in and out. If your tongue arches up try to keep it relaxed. You can control the air

Positive Flow Childbirth

flow with either the teeth or the tongue, or a combination of both. But again, try to keep the tongue as relaxed as possible.

Find the way of controlling the air flow that feels most relaxed to you. If none are relaxed then you might do it one way for a period of time and then switch to a different position. The important thing is to make it so comfortable that it doesn't distract you from the other things that we will be talking about.

Our goal is to have long slow breaths. The longer and slower the better. We do not want to do this with short breaths. Short breaths do not lead to the level of inner withdrawal that we are seeking. They also increase the chances of lightheadedness: especially with beginners.

When you practice this start with just 3 to 5 minutes. Don't go any longer at first. It is better to increase the length of the breath up to the count of 12 or more with intensity and concentration than the total amount of time. If you start to get light headed you will need to breathe more slowly and practice for a shorter length of time.

You can practice the Hong-Sau technique before and/ or after practicing the pranayama technique. Don't forget to include periods of sitting in the silence. Gently look up into the spiritual eye and rest inwardly connected to peace, calmness and joy.

Over a period of 6 to 8 months you should work up to a period 30 minutes continuous pranayama practice. Again, inner focus and longer controlled breaths are very important. You also need to stay relaxed.

Now for the hard part!

It isn't just the moving of the breath that we are attempting here. We want to control the prana - life force - in the body as well. As you inhale, feel that there is a gentle current of energy rising up the center of your body in the inner spine. Start at the base of the spine and feel this energy climb slowly up towards the brain and then stopping at the spiritual eye during the 3 count hold. In the beginning feel that you are consciously drawing the energy up the spine through the breath, but eventually we want to be so mentally identified with the energy that it begins to feel like the upward flow of energy is causing the breath to flow.

You must be relaxed and receptive to feel this inner energy flow. Use utmost attention but without physical or mental tension. In the beginning you can try to visualize the energy until you start to feel it. It isn't a static feeling, it is a flow. This flow of energy as it moves up and down the spine can create a powerful magnetism. Thus we return to the idea of spiritually magnetizing ourselves so that we can perceive Spirit.

As the inner spine becomes magnetized our consciousness is pulled within. We detach ourselves from sense attachments and begin to live from our true center in Spirit. It is this experience of calm interiorization that will tell you if you are doing the technique correctly. If it just seems like huffing and puffing and you don't feel any different after practicing it, then you don't have it right. Pay close attention to how you are practicing the technique and then refer carefully again to the instructions. Again, I encourage person-to-person instruction when possible.

There are many techniques in the yoga teachings that are variations on the same basic technique that we have just discussed. Some are more or less effective than others by the nature of the technique itself, but most important to the usefulness of any technique is the quality and then the quantity of the effort that is applied to its use. Some people can effectively use these techniques after a few weeks or months while others will need years to master them sufficiently for use in childbirth.

Positive Flow Childbirth

Where you fit in this equation can only be judged by yourself. I can only say that these techniques are fully capable of giving you the results that you need for childbirth if you master them. Let your own experiments be the test of this truth. Practice them and see for yourself!

Now that we have discussed the basic techniques, let's see how they are actually applied during the birth.

Chapter 23

Relax, Withdraw & Climb the Mountain

There are three basic stages to the labor process. Let's go through them and see how we can best use our various techniques.

The first stage begins when you know that the labor process has begun. Your medical team will be guiding you in understanding what to watch for. The best thing you can do during this time is to stay quiet and calm. Let nature take its course. Take a moment and pray for God's blessing on you and your child. Give all worries to God. Visualize yourself resting in the all-comforting hands of the universal Divine Mother.

During this time you can do anything that you feel comfortable doing. The key here is distraction. Stay busy enough so that you are not drawn into anxiety or excessive body consciousness, but not so busy that you become mentally agitated. Read a book, listen to calming music, have a friendly conversation, rock in a rocking chair, anything that feels comfortable. There is no way of knowing how long this is going to take so pace yourself.

You can practice meditation for a few minutes at a time to keep yourself centered but don't overdo it, you want to save your intensity for the birth. Just stay relaxed and inwardly calm.

Positive Flow Childbirth

When the contractions become so intense that simple distractions and/or a few deep breaths won't do the job anymore you will want to move into the labor room if you aren't already there. Keep in mind that you don't know how long the labor process will take. So you don't want to jump the gun with intense inward efforts, at the same time you don't want to wait so long that you can't disconnect from the pain. This is a judgment call that only you can make.

Having made the decision, now is the time to begin using our techniques for withdrawing from body consciousness. Practice Hong-Sau for a few minutes and then begin your practice of pranayama. Take it slowly and easily. Don't be in a rush. There should still be plenty of time between contractions for you to apply your concentration towards withdrawing from body consciousness.

As contractions come accept them. Let the energy of the contraction feed your inner concentration. Transmute the sensations by drawing them into the spine and up to the spiritual eye. The more that you have prepared yourself before the birth by regular practice the easier and more effective this will be. As you draw the energy up and down the spine feel yourself becoming more and more inwardly focused and connected to your heart center. Let that become your center of awareness and do your pranayama from that perspective.

If the discomfort of the contractions pulls you out of this inner awareness there is another thing that you can do. Use the double breath that we use for the energization exercise. The short and long inhalation through the nose, followed by a short and long exhalation through the mouth. Don't tense the body while you use the double breath. Instead feel that the power of your breath is dissipating the pain. Feel that your conscious breath control is above and on top of the pain. Use this during the contractions only as necessary. As soon as the contraction is completed go back into the spine using your pranayama. The more withdrawn you can become the more effective this will be. I can't stress this enough: The interiorization of the mind away from the body consciousness is the most effective thing that you can do.

Another thing that you can do if things get tough is to laugh. I don't mean losing control laughing, but keep your sense of humor. In a subtle way this laughing at the pain keeps you above it. Always stay inwardly focused, connected to the heart and spiritual eye. If you experiment with other techniques, try to stay inwardly connected to peace and calmness. Practice sitting in the silence between contractions if you need a rest from the pranayama. The more successful you have been with your pranayama practice, the more inwardly disconnected from the pain you will be.

Once the cervix is dilated sufficiently, it will be time to change tactics. This is a very sensitive time because if you have been successful in withdrawing from the body consciousness it will take an act of will to now enter back into the body. Sensitive coaching is essential at this stage.

In most cases the baby isn't going to come out unless you help. So you will need to direct your mind back to a greater body awareness. This is where the analogy of climbing a mountain comes in. At some point in a long difficult ascent there is a decision to push for the top. At that point it is no holds barred. You must take every ounce of strength and determination that you have and go for it.

That is what this third stage is all about: going for it! You are almost at the peak so grasp your God given determination and feel the Divine power flowing through you. Use the same principles that we learned in the energization exercises.

Positive Flow Childbirth

Consciously send the energy to your muscles as you push. Under the direction of the medical staff you will be told when to push. Feel that the life force is entering your body through the medulla and powering up the muscles. You can use a double breath inhalation before you push and the double breath exhalation afterwards. Use your pranayama breath between pushing, but maintain your connection to the physical process now, you need to be fully present and not withdrawn.

It is essential that you enter into this final phase completely. Don't let your mind fly away because you are tired. Don't let doubt creep in. You are a child of God and as His child the power of the universe can come to your aid. Call upon Him for your strength and He will be with you.

Chapter 24

Coaching

The best coach you can get will probably be your mate, but things don't always work out that way. If they don't then choose your helper carefully. It must be a person who you can count on to be there. No ifs, ands, or buts. They must be there!

The coach should be someone whom you are confident won't fall apart once things start happening. Of course you will have your medical help so you won't be without additional support, but you don't want to be worrying about your coach. That's the one person who's only task is seeing to your needs.

The coach should be completely in tune with your approach to the birth and if you plan on using anything in this book the coach needs to read it as well. Whatever breathing techniques you use the coach will need to be completely familiar with them. Also the coach should go with you to any educational classes that you attend.

Spend as much time as possible meditating with your coach in the months before the birth so that you feel a oneness in the harmony of Spirit. This time together before the birth will help you to develop an inner connection that wasn't there before. With this deepening sense of attunement your coach will begin to empathize with your changing condition like no other person. Through this empathy your coach may begin to intuit your needs instead of needing to ask or be asked. This sense of oneness will give you an added feeling of confidence and encouragement. It also provides a buffer so that you don't have to be distracted by other things going on around you.

If you plan on using the internalized approach that I am sharing with you then the coach must understand exactly what you are trying to do and if necessary try to prevent people or events from pulling you out of your withdrawn state until the right time. Once it is time to push then your coach will be your guide back into the body by encouraging you to make the transition.

One of the best ways for the coach to stay with the mother is to do the breathing right alongside her. When Bhavani started her pranayama I was with her doing every breath. We flowed in a kind of unison that gave a greater depth to her internalization. She knew I was right with her and that gave her the confidence to keep going deeper and deeper. Our combined magnetism took her deeper than she could have gone by herself. This kind of support can make all the difference. But the coach will have to be willing to put in the preparation time to be really affective.

It is also important that your medical help completely understand what you are trying to do. Most midwives and doctors are used to talking and touching, suggesting a massage here and there, trying to be generally helpful - after all that is what they think they are there for. Once a person starts to go within all of that attention can be distracting and defeats the mother's attempts to withdraw. When our midwife couldn't help herself and wanted to massage Bhavani I knew it wasn't the right thing to do, so I gave her a silent no with my head and she got the message. This kind of thing will depend on the ability of the mother to withdraw. If mental withdrawal from the senses isn't happening then of course massage or anything else you want to try is fine. It is essential that these issues be discussed with the midwife ahead of time.

This flexibility is very important and the coach needs to help evaluate how things are going. If mother is doing fine then protect her space. But if she isn't focused and is spacing out in some way then you need to react with confidence and clarity. Having a bag of tricks for every situation is one of the things that the medical help can offer. If what you have planned isn't working then let the professionals give suggestions. There is no question that giving birth to a child is an adventure, so take it in that spirit and be flexible: Go with the flow!

The coach should not be responsible for taking pictures, videos or any other responsibility that might distract from helping the mother. Careful planning ahead of time will save much confusion during the birth. Mother and coach should spend plenty of time discussing every aspect of the birth so that every imaginable contingency is thought through in advance. This type of thoroughness is not just practical, but it is the correct use of our God-given intelligence.

As a part of supporting the mother the coach should do everything possible to maintain the highest vibration in the room. It is easy for people to get excited at these times and the energy can swing in either a positive or a negative direction. Don't allow negative energies to develop between any of the people in attendance.

And above all, keep the thought of God's presence ever alive. Keep drawing on the heavenly energies to guide and protect.

Chapter 25

Plan Ahead

When the time finally comes for the birth the months of anticipation will bring about an intense focusing of your energies on the moment. It is best to have planned every aspect of the birth ahead of time so that you can be relaxed and fully embrace the experience.

If you are having the birth at a hospital or birthing center then you won't have to think about medical supplies for the birth itself. If you are having the baby at home you will want to review everything that will be needed with your medical support person. Consider not only the birth, but anything that you might need for a couple of weeks following the birth.

Everything should be ready to go at least 6 or 8 weeks in advance of the due date. There are a lot of things that you don't think of until you really put your mind to it, so here is just a partial list of things to consider. Also consult with others for more ideas.

Attendees: Who will attend the birth and what will they do while they are waiting? Who will be in the room with you during the birth and who will be nearby in another room? Who will contact friends and family not in attendance to keep them apprised of the situation? Will you want the phone to ring during the birth if you are at home? Make sure it is clear to everyone what type of environment you want to have during the birth.

Atmosphere: What kind of environment do you want to create? If you are going to try and withdraw inwardly you will want it quiet as possible. Do you want pictures, candles or other special items? Do what you can to be sure that the air in the room will be fresh. What about pictures and video? Consider who will do this and how it will affect the energy in the room.

Food: Food will be needed for before, during and after the birth for everyone in attendance. There is no way of knowing exactly how long it will take. It is always a good idea to freeze some meals so you don't have to cook right after the birth. Friends can help with this too.

Clothes: What clothes will you wear during the birth and afterwards? Don't let the birth catch you with all of your clothes in the laundry! This can be a messy process, so have plenty of changes on hand. You probably won't want to get up and do laundry for awhile!

Baby Stuff: What type of diapers are you going to use? Have plenty on hand! Blankets. Clothes. Preparations for bottle feeding just in case breast feeding doesn't work out for you. Where will the baby sleep?

Emergencies: Along with the physical preparations you will need to plan for emergencies if you are at home. How will mother and/or child get to the closest hospital if needed. If the delivery is upstairs how will Mom get downstairs? Will Dad carry her? If only the child or the mother need extra medical assistance who will go with whom? Is a vehicle available with gas and the route known to the driver? Or will you call 911? You may even want to check out the local hospital in advance so there aren't any hitches should you need to go there.

Positive Flow Childbirth

Medical Issues: There are also many medical issues that should be considered in advance. They are not pleasant to think about but making as clear a decision as you can in advance is very helpful. How do you feel about life support? If the doctor must choose the life of the child or the mother, who do you choose?

Earlier we talked about how there isn't just one right answer to many of these issues. While some would say that the mother should offer her life for the child, that isn't always for the greatest good. Remember the sailor in the boat who could do more good by staying around to help others? I'm not saying it should be one way or the other, I'm just saying don't jump to conclusions without giving it considerable thought and meditation. Carefully go through all of the potential problems with your medical staff and make sure that they understand your wishes. Search your deepest feelings and try to feel God's guidance.

From a spiritual point of view our responsibility is to do our very best, align ourselves with the positive flow of life and give the results to God. We don't often know if the choices that we make in life are the best ones. But whatever happens, even when we make mistakes it can be turned into good by keeping our motives as selfless as possible while always striving to improve our attunement to the will of God.

We don't want to cloud the birth experience with fears. So once you have made your decisions set them aside. Immerse yourself in the thought of God's protective presence. Feel the joy of life's positive flow and surround yourself in the light of Spirit. These positive thoughts will strengthen your magnetism and lessen the possibility of problems.

If you have done your homework, by preparing mentally, physically, and spiritually to the best of your ability, then you have done your part. Now you can move forward with confidence to one of life's greatest moments: the birth of a child. Savor this experience. Though it be physically and mentally challenging the rewards are truly great.

Chapter 26

Putting it All Together

Now that we have discussed most of the major aspects of the birth and the spiritual principles behind them let's put it all together. In order to do that we could create a hypothetical situation but I feel that you will get more of the inspiration of the experience if we tell a true story. So I will tell you about the birth of my own children.

While we take this journey together, remember I'm not saying that we did it the ultimate way or that the way we did it is the way you should do it. I hope that you will use this example as a springboard to create your own view of what is best for you. Keep in mind the many principles underneath the actions that we have discussed. Then determine for yourself how they can best be applied to your situation.

I should mention that we based our decisions on our many years of following our spiritual path. These years of regular meditation and other spiritual practices gave us a perspective that may be different from yours. Your decisions and abilities will depend to some degree on what practices you have been using for your ongoing spiritual upliftment. It also can depend on your natural strength of mind. You may be more able or less able than Bhavani to control your energies during the birth process. Only you can evaluate whether or not you can handle labor with the techniques that we have discussed.

So as you explore the possibilities make sure that you balance your ideal with what you really think you can handle. I want to re-emphasize that there is no conflict of energies if you use additional techniques during the birth that we did not use. The key is to do what works for you, not what you wish would work! If you have any doubts about your ability to use the pranayama technique to withdraw from the senses or if for any other physical or mental reason you are in doubt then learn a widely used birthing technique to use as back up.

When evaluating these techniques I would simply say choose one that is proven to work and that seems most in tune with the principles of staying calm and inwardly focused. And remember, using a non-spiritually based technique doesn't make it unspiritual. For any technique to work at all it must in some way use the same energy that we have been talking about. The difference, as I mentioned before, is that most widely used breathing techniques tend to work from the outside in rather than the inside out. They also don't take into account the deeper energies in the spine that we have talked about. But that doesn't make them "bad".

You can use all of the other ideas that we have discussed and just have these other birthing techniques available to help if necessary. I wouldn't call that "unspiritual". I'd call it prudent.

So now, let's take a journey together. It is the story about a couple who tried to have a child and got two instead. Isn't life full of surprises!

Chapter 27

From the Beginning

Bhavani and I had been friends for a number of years before we became a couple. But as soon as we did get together we knew that we would have a child. For some it is a question that must be carefully weighed with pros and cons. For us it was a natural expansion of our love.

As I mentioned earlier, Bhavani, had two children from a previous marriage: Cristi who was then ten years old and Daniel who was twelve. When Bhavani had labored with Daniel and Cristi she just followed the doctor's orders and had always regretted letting the hospital personnel take control of her the way that they did. At the time she just didn't realize that she had a choice. This time she determined she would make choices consciously.

Suffice to say that we in our own way managed to conceive a child. Each couple must choose for themselves how, when and where it is most appropriate. The important thing about style is that it be vibrationally as high as possible. We endeavored to do our best in that regard.

It was on a pleasant afternoon in the garden when Bhavani had that experience where she felt the souls enter her body. She didn't tell me right away. But some weeks later when the pregnancy was confirmed she did tell me; though she didn't say anything about being confused that she felt so much energy. In retrospect we both agree that she didn't really want to know at that point that it was twins! Needless to say I was ecstatic!

As I look back at the many decisions that we made over the ensuing months I realize that we really had very few discussions. I don't think that it would be the same for everyone. We just seemed to see things the same way. That doesn't make us better or worse than other couples, it just makes it a little easier. If an issue needs to be discussed, then by all means discuss away.

One thing that I noticed is that at each step of the way when a new direction needed to be taken the doors would open. This I attribute to our sense of harmony with the positive flow of life.

That we wanted to have the birth at home was never in question, so we began to search for the help that we would need right away. We were referred by a friend to a midwife who lived some 15 miles away and so we went to see her. It is somewhat awkward for me to admit, after telling you to consider carefully who you choose for medical help, that as soon as we met Miriam we knew that she was the one for us. Not only did she answer all of our questions with no hurry, but she exuded a feeling that just felt right. As soon as we walked out of her office Bhavani and I smiled at each other. We didn't even have to say: This is a person we can trust.

Having never been through this process before I have to say I was much more eager than Bhavani. She seemed totally unconcerned with most of the information in the classes that Miriam gave to all of her expectant mothers. I think we only attended one or two out of eight. Bhavani just said that she already knew where babies come from and left it at that.

Positive Flow Childbirth

We did discuss with Miriam at much length the various conditions that might prevent us from having the birth at home. Miriam spoke frankly about the kinds of situations that she was or was not willing to handle. Her honesty and clear explanations of the details gave us even more confidence in our choice. Here was a person who knew what she could or couldn't handle.

Since I wanted to receive the child with my own hands as it emerged into the world I gave special attention to the physical details that she discussed. Remember, we still didn't know it was twins!

For the first two trimesters we drove together once a month to see Miriam. At each visit, along with generally checking Bhavani over, Miriam would measure the fundal height of the abdomen. This distance can help to give an indication of when the birth will take place. Because of this measurement and the fact that careful listening with the stethoscope found only one heartbeat we were informed that the birth was one month advanced from the date that we believed to be correct. This didn't fit with what Bhavani and I knew from our physical relationship to be true, as well as, not fitting the date that she had felt the soul coming into the body. We really didn't know what to think, so we just took a wait and see attitude.

During one of our visits to see Miriam she asked Bhavani if she was going to take a class in breathing techniques for the labor. Bhavani simply replied that she didn't think that it would be necessary. Over the next few visits Miriam asked again about taking classes but each time Bhavani declined. I never entered into this discussion. I always felt that it was Bhavani's decision. After all, she was the one having the baby!

Truthfully, I must admit I was a little concerned about it. When you have never actually tried something, even if you believe it will work, there is still that sense of never before having done it. But I knew Bhavani to be an extremely capable person so I let it rest.

It might seem to some that her attitude was somewhat cavalier. But actually, she had been doing for years the very things that would make the birth as easy as possible. She meditated daily. She not only practiced Hatha yoga daily but she taught several classes a week until the beginning of the ninth month. She daily practiced the Kriya yoga pranayama technique. These weren't things that she did for the birth, they had been a regular part of her life for many years; so it was unnecessary to add them because of the pregnancy.

After 6 months the visits to Miriam were stepped up to every other week. Wouldn't you know it that at one of the few visits that I wasn't able to attend, Bhavani got the shock of her life. Miriam was listening for the baby's heartbeat and found more than one. Suddenly Miriam's measurements made sense. The date that we believed to be right was correct. Bhavani's size was larger not because of the date, but because there were twins!

There was now only six weeks to go. And we just found out we were having twins. Would Miriam still do the delivery at home? What new problems could arise? What would the solutions be? Suddenly a thousand new questions and all because of TWINS!

Chapter 28

Adjusting to New Horizons

It was a few hours after Bhavani's visit with Miriam that I came home. As soon as I saw Bhavani I knew something was wrong. When I asked her what was up she hesitated for a moment. My mind started to race with unpleasant possibilities. She looked at me and then she burst into tears as she blurted out, "Twins!"

Everyone has probably had something happen in their life that is so unexpected that for a moment your brain just shuts down and stops. Well, that's what mine was doing while I hugged my sobbing wife. It was the only time in the whole process that I ever saw her evenness of mind and emotions waiver.

I knew immediately that it wasn't a rejection of the souls that had come to us but a culmination of the pressures that were building up inside. Not only was she now having a child after her thirty-fifth birthday, but there were two of them! The thought of what that entailed was just momentarily overwhelming and she vented her feelings with enthusiasm. As I comforted her, I on the other hand became very excited. I thought that it was great! The more the merrier!

While we have discussed the value of transmuting sensations and emotions into the spine and up, there are times when we just have to let them out. The suppression of feelings is not the goal of the spiritual life. If the energy contained in a feeling cannot be turned inward and positively transmuted, then as long as it won't cause harm to another person it should be vented. This was a case where Bhavani's feelings needed to come out. After a short period of adjustment, like several days, she finally came to grips with the abundance that God was bringing us.

On several of our trips to Miriam's it was suggested to Bhavani that she eat more. Bhavani took the time to explain to Miriam that she always ate what her body told her to eat and that she could do only that. Some years previous Bhavani had her gall bladder removed, as a result she had to be especially careful about what she ate.

The practice of listening to your body's needs is very much a part of living in harmony with the body. Many people don't realize that the food we eat isn't just proteins, fats and carbohydrates: it is consciousness. It has vibrations that give a quality of consciousness to the food. By paying attention to this we can eat foods that are not only good for the cells of the body, but good for the soul. That's the root meaning of soul food - food that has been prepared with love, like the food from a loving mother. It carries a vibration that feeds the soul and not just the body. As long as I have known Bhavani she has always approached eating this way and she is rarely ill.

As soon as Bhavani recovered from the shock of carrying two babies instead of one we scheduled another appointment with Miriam. The biggest question was: Would we still be able to have the babies at home? I don't mind saying that I was concerned. I had a strong desire to have the birth at home. I wanted to receive the children with my own hands and I didn't think a hospital would allow me to do that.

Positive Flow Childbirth

At our meeting with Miriam we found that she had delivered twins at home before, but she was concerned about the position of the babies. If they were both breach - feet first - she wouldn't do it. If one was breach, she might. If they were both head first, since everything else was going smoothly, she would be willing.

The next step was to have a sonogram done. Normally we wouldn't have chosen to do this, but for the sake of having the babies at home we decided to. I am told that the sonogram does no harm to the child or mother, but I don't always believe what I am told. In any case, we decided that it was worth the risk, so we had it done at our local hospital. The resultant picture showed that both babies were head down.

From the picture it was clear how one was behind the other. It was because the one in the front had dropped a little in preparation for the birth that the heartbeat of the one behind had become audible. It wasn't clear from the picture what the sexes were. And it was just as well because it was our personal preference that we didn't want to know. There wasn't any great spiritual reason for this, it was just our preference. Now that we knew the position of the babies Miriam gave the okay and it was a GO for home delivery.

Needless to say, we had to double up on many of the provisions that had been gathered weeks ago. We also needed to work out the logistics of another child at the birth. It added many more possibilities for which we needed to be prepared. It was like doing the logistics for an ascent of Mt. Everest. We planned everything to the last detail. If this happens, then we do this. If that happens, than we do that.

Through all of this preparation Bhavani continued everyday to meditate and do her yoga postures. While she was sometimes very tired, she never complained and always was quick to smile. This is the fruit of the spiritual life - a natural grace during times of challenge. She had been given more than she bargained for but she was embracing it with a smile.

It isn't that anyone who complains or expresses discomfort is unspiritual. We are all spiritual by the fact that we are manifestations of God. But each person must decide and then act upon their desire to live in harmony with Spirit. To the extent that we are successful in those efforts we will be able to express the joy of Spirit even under trying circumstances.

As the eagerly awaited time approached we continued to make our final preparations.

Chapter 29

Ready, Set, Go!

The extent to which we prepared for the birth of the twins is worthy of note if for no other reason than to impress upon you your responsibility to do everything that you can to help things go well. It isn't good enough to sit in the corner and pray that God will take care of things. We need to be His active instruments by doing as much as we can.

Now that we were expecting two little ones we had to escalate our efforts. We had originally planned for two midwives to be in attendance; one for mother and another for child. Now we needed three midwives. We also had separate sets of sterile instruments for each, as well as anything else that the midwives thought they could possibly use: including oxygen.

Since we were planning to have the birth upstairs we had a portable stretcher just in case I wasn't able or there to carry Bhavani downstairs if she needed to go to the hospital. Each midwife was assigned to a person. Miriam to Bhavani and the others to a child each. If someone had to go to the hospital I would drive the midwife and patient to the hospital. Then I would return to the house. Since we lived only about a mile from the hospital this seemed acceptable. Those at home could always call 911 in a pinch.

We arranged a phone tree so that all it would take was one call out of our house to inform our family and friends. And we requested them not to call us but to wait for word.

Now it seems so simple, but as you make all of these preparations each one takes thought and time. Make sure that you don't wait until the last minute. Those little guys come early sometimes!

We had a long discussion with Daniel and Cristi about attending the birth. There is much to be said about being present during a birth. We discussed with them frankly the pros and cons. At first they had much enthusiasm for it, but as they began to understand more realistically what it would be like watching the business end of a birth, well, that initial interest began to dwindle. In the end it wasn't the potential for blood that swung their vote. They decided that they would feel very uncomfortable if they saw their mother in pain.

These issues should be carefully discussed, taking into account the age of the child. It is a very dramatic moment and can leave an impression for a lifetime. Should a child be attendant at the birth there should be an adult whose sole responsibility is to care for the child. The adult responsible for the child needs to be capable of dealing with any feelings that might arise in the child; including the need to leave quickly. If there is more than one child, at least one adult in the birthing room and one adult outside to greet anyone who needs to leave would be the minimum coverage. You don't want mom to be distracted by children.

Make sure that there are extra sheets for the birthing bed. And double check that there won't be any problems with heating or cooling the house. If it is winter you will want to make sure the house is sufficiently warm, and in summer sufficiently cool.

Positive Flow Childbirth

You will come up with more little details that need to be taken care of the longer you think about it. Making a list and checking it twice isn't only for Christmas. And speaking of Christmas, it was December 21st at about 9 pm when the fabled stork began to ring our doorbell.

So with Daniel and Cristi off to Grandma's we began this great event by beginning to draw our attention within, away from the world and all its affairs, away from doubts and lists and concerns of any kind. We drew silently within where we could feel closer to our Heavenly Father and our Divine Mother.

Chapter 30

Unto us,
Two Children
are Born!

Once the contractions started we sat for a while until we were sure this was it. Then I placed a call to Miriam and let her know it was happening. After that I really lost track of time until the birth itself. And then I was only aware of the time because, as we had planned, someone had called out the time of the first birth.

Bhavani and I just sat quietly in the living room, sharing the beginning of this very special moment. After some time we started the very natural to us process of going deep within ourselves. By the time Miriam arrived we had gone upstairs to the bedroom. Bhavani was lying on the bed propped up by a few pillows. I sat next to her on the bed holding her hand. We were practicing our pranayama. I don't remember letting Miriam in, so I think that she found her own way upstairs. My next clear memory is of her checking to see how far along Bhavani was. I knew that I had to be Bhavani's bridge with Miriam so I tried to maintain enough outward awareness to deal with questions while keeping withdrawn enough inside to be attuned to Bhavani.

Miriam was very sensitive to our quietness and didn't intrude any more than necessary. Every once in a while she would come in, check on us, and then leave. While she was gone I would watch Bhavani's breath and match mine to it.

It became clear that Bhavani was riding the energy of the contractions with a very inward focus. As Bhavani drew smooth continuous deep breaths fully focused on the energy within she exhibited no signs of discomfort. She hardly moved her body at all. She was fully withdrawn.

I was careful not to move so that I wouldn't disturb her and I talked as quietly as possible when Miriam had a question. I think that what we were doing was so unusual for Miriam, even though we had explained what we were going to do, that she couldn't quite believe it was working. Convinced that she must be needed for something she offered to massage Bhavani. As she made the offer I watched Bhavani's face. Her eyes were closed but she nodded a slow no. I knew she didn't want to be touched so I advised Miriam against it. When the soul withdraws into the spine time ceases to matter and the only reality is the oneness of the soul as Spirit.

Only later upon reflection did I realize how deep I had gone and thus all the deeper Bhavani had gone. As I think about it, I realize that nothing was really done outwardly except checking for the dilation of the cervix until it was time to push. Once Miriam gave the word that it was time, I began to gently pull Bhavani back into the body. I started quietly at first and then more firmly talking to her. I encouraged her to come back out because it was time to push.

It took a few minutes for Bhavani to make the transition. At first it seemed like she was reluctant, but gradually she started to respond. I had the impression that she was thinking: But why? It's so nice in here!

It is important to remember not to rush this process of coming back into the body. But once you start keep it coming at a steady pace. As I held Bhavani's hand I squeezed it with gradually firmer pressure to get her attention. Once Bhavani started actively to come back she firmly took hold of herself and went to work.

At this point, because the baby is very low in the birth canal, you don't want it to take any longer than necessary. It gets a little tight in there so you have to stay with it until the job is done, no matter how long it takes.

Miriam continuously monitored Bhavani's and the babies' heartbeats. All three midwives were now in the room and we were ready for the final phase. Once it is time to push there seems to be a flow that will be different for everyone. One of the advantages of home birth is that you can go with this flow, where as in the hospital your space is limited.

After pushing for some time while on the bed Miriam informed Bhavani that she wasn't making sufficient progress. She suggested that Bhavani get up off the bed and let gravity help. So Bhavani got up and started experimenting with different standing and squatting positions. She used the double breath to inhale and then tensed and pushed for all she was worth. I was fully impressed! At one point she was standing there all on her own, just like I had imagined the American Indian women did, no cries of pain, no muss or fuss, just getting down to business.

Some women throw up during labor. Needing to relieve the bowels and/or the bladder is even more common. There is something about the relaxing of the muscles at that time that can help things along. After trying standing positions and then trying the bed again Bhavani decided that she had to relieve her bladder. As I was holding her hand at the time she took me with her. I tried to mind my own business, while she did hers.

Well, the process of relaxing seemed to do the trick for her. Suddenly, with surprise in her voice I heard Bhavani say: It's coming! I immediately got in behind Bhavani as she stood up, to help support her while Miriam moved in to have a look. Miriam said she could see the top of the head and asked Bhavani if she could make it to the bed. Bhavani didn't answer, she just pushed for all she was worth.

So here we were in the bathroom, very tight quarters, and Bhavani was partially squatting and mostly leaning back on me. I grabbed her around the torso with my left arm and supported us with my right arm against the wall. We were both leaning back at about a sixty degree angle. Suddenly, instead of receiving the child I was underneath Bhavani almost as if I were also having the child. Her hips were pressed against my legs, my stomach against her lower back, and I could feel the fluctuating tension in her abdominal muscles. It was a totally unexpected turn of events!

As the baby started to emerge Miriam looked up at me, knowing that I wasn't going to fulfill my desire to receive the child. But I just smiled at her and said: Go for it. As Bhavani and I, head to head, watched the first little one come out I was surprised to see how clean and fresh it looked. Often babies come out looking a little worse for wear.

We could soon see that it was a girl and then that magic moment arrived. There is nothing else quite like it. Miriam quickly cleaned out the mouth and then without a cry, just a little gasp, that first breath pronounced complete arrival.

She was here with us. A baby girl at 2:45 a.m. December 22, 1981.

Miriam cut the umbilical cord and handed our daughter to the midwife who was assigned to check her out. We moved back to the bed and Bhavani relaxed for a few minutes propped up on the pillows the way we had started. After confirming that our little girl was healthy she was wrapped up and held by

Bhavani and I for a few minutes. But, as joyous as that moment was, we weren't done yet!

During this time Miriam constantly monitored Bhavani's condition. It seemed like just a few minutes had passed and then we were back at it for baby number two.

Again Bhavani searched for just the right position. She went through all of the previously tried positions and none of them worked. Finally we all looked at each other and said in unison: Back to the bathroom!

You have to go with where it is happening! And the bathroom is where both of our kids wanted to be born. And as I think about it, two souls so close that they would come as twins would certainly want to start in the same place. So again, I was behind Bhavani and going through it with her. It was such a unique perspective. I mean I wasn't having the baby but I couldn't get much closer to feeling that I was in any other position. As Bhavani pushed I mentally pushed. I tried to feel our oneness both in body and soul. It was an amazing experience.

Once we got things going in the bathroom it didn't take long. And suddenly, as if we weren't expecting it, there was another head peeking out into an unfamiliar world. Again I was struck by how clean and pink the face was. With a final push at 3:10 a.m. to go with our little daughter we now had a son. He used a louder voice with his first breath, but never a cry. Maybe he wanted to make sure that we knew he was here!

I can only think that Bhavani's deep state of calmness throughout the birth was strong enough to provide the reassurance to the little ones that everything was going to be fine. For they both were calm and quiet, perfectly happy. And so were their parents.

Chapter 31

Rejoice!

No matter whether things go smoothly or with great difficulty, remember that all of life is God's gift to us. Even our most difficult trials are blessed opportunities to grow towards our home in Spirit. This is a truth that many people don't understand, which causes them to question how God could even exist since there is so much suffering in this world. This world is truly a fire in which the kinks of our character are straightened out, as if being worked on by a heavenly forge.

The thing to remember is that we have drawn to ourselves everything we experience in this life by our past actions even if we can't remember those circumstances. And the quality of energy that we are currently putting out towards the challenges that we face determines what effect these current experiences will have on our future.

All experiences in life, both pleasant and unpleasant, should be used to feed the fire of our desire to know God more fully. There are countless stories about how the saints have turned terrible suffering into joyous communion with God. And not enough stories of people using their joy to feed their spiritual fervor. So take the exhaustion, the joy and any other emotions that you feel after the birth into yourself and offer them up to God. Let the intensity of the experience deepen your awareness that God is the source of all experiences.

After the twins were born Bhavani and I rested while we cuddled our little bundles of joy. During this time Miriam continued to monitor Bhavani and the children.

Sometime after the birth the placenta will pass from the uterus. This is a sensitive time because if the walls of the uterus are torn then bleeding can become a problem. Apparently this had happened with Bhavani and the midwives began to confer as to how much bleeding was going to be acceptable. One was of the opinion that it might be time to take Bhavani for further medical attention. Another felt that we could wait a little longer. Miriam did what she could to help the situation and then we waited. In times like this we should place our attention strongly at the spiritual eye and pray deeply that God's Will be done.

The key is to be detached while focusing our energy as a channel for positive blessings towards the situation. Unless you feel specifically guided to pray for a particular outcome it is better to stay a neutral positive force for the highest good that is in tune to the Will of God. So in this spirit, as we rested I mentally sent energy to Bhavani's uterus. After about 20 or 30 minutes Miriam gave us the nod that everything was going to be alright. We then fully relaxed into the immensity of our success and good fortune.

If you have never attended a birth you haven't yet experienced the full dimension of the occasion. Reading about it or seeing it on video doesn't fully communicate the wondrous qualities of energy that surround the moment. There is an elemental universal presence that connects that moment in time to the beginnings of the creation itself. I have never had any experience in my life that more communicated the miracle of life.

Positive Flow Childbirth

Our lives so often seem dull and mundane, filled with the monotonous details of daily existence. When we connect ourselves to the spark of life that animates us then everything is changed. Suddenly we can see that life is full of infinite potential; unlimited possibilities!

Now that we had climbed the mountain of birth we were to begin an even greater challenge, that of living up to the trust in which God had placed us. These two souls would look to us not only for physical sustenance, but for guidance, patience and soul nurturing love.

Our hearts were full of the love that God gave us, that we might make it larger by sharing it with these two souls. We did fully rejoice in the moment.

Chapter 32

What's in a Name?

Many people are given a name out of love and respect for a relative. Others are given names that sound nice or evoke an image that is pleasant to the parents. Some like names that rhyme with the last name. Others get the name that their parents wish they had gotten. So, what's in a name?

Once again it is helpful to go back to the basics. This world is a manifestation of vibration. The bible says: In the beginning was the word and the word was with God and the word was God. All of the creation is vibrating with the manifested presence of God. In the Christian tradition this is also called the Holy Ghost. It is described as thunder and trumpets, and the sound of many waters. In India the word that is used for this universal sound is AUM (sounds like om).

Because we are all manifestations of this universal principle our own bodies put out a vibration. It is most easily perceived as one's aura - which is a combination of light emanations that come from each person's astral body. Some people can see auras but most of us cannot see them. What's important about this is that our vibration is the story of where we have been and our actions today determine where our lives will go.

Positive Flow Childbirth

Earlier we discussed how music can affect our vibration, that we should only listen to music that is uplifting. This outward influence on us is just as real as the positive effect of good food or as the negative effect of negative environments. When we call someone's name we are speaking an affirmation of their vibration. We are giving them energy and the name itself has the ability to enhance the positive vibrations that we want to feel and send when we think of someone. If you call someone Dumpy they are certainly going to be more likely to feel dumpy, then if you call them Happy.

So when we give someone a name it should be an affirmation of the attitude or vibration that we want for them. If you want your son to be a great sportsman then try calling him Sport or Champ. Or name him after a great sportsman that you hope he will emulate. That will reinforce the attitude you are trying to support. If you want your daughter to develop grace then you might call her Grace: likewise for Hope or Joy.

The one thing that I would caution against are names that seem cute in the beginning but cause children much grief when they go to school. Children are notorious for twisting names into torment for an innocent child.

When we were seeking names for the twins I spent much time meditating on the subject. I wanted the names not only to fit their vibrations but to inspire them towards the best future that I could wish for them. For me that meant the names had to be spiritually based. It is interesting that as we discussed names before we knew about having twins I came up with a boy's name and a girl's name. Bhavani and I agreed on the names so we thought we were set. Then when we found out about having twins I tried to come up with two more names; in case it was two girls or two boys. As hard as I tried I couldn't come up with any more names! Finally we just decided that we would have to wait until after the birth to decide. We had no idea it would work out the way it did.

Coming up with the name is partly intellectual and partly intuitional. We wanted names that would reflect our spiritual path which is a blending of Eastern and Western philosophies. So we decided on giving each child a Western name and an Eastern name. Then came the task of choosing from any number of names that could fit in those broad categories.

Here I applied principles that we have already discussed. With concentration I tried to put myself inwardly in the positive flow that was right for the children. I didn't rush the process. I regularly broadcast inwardly the mental message of need and waited with patience. I took up the habit of mentally asking and then listening for an answer. I got quite used to not hearing anything! But I didn't give up. Then over a period of about a week the names started to present themselves.

First were the Christian names. There was Theresa and Francis. Theresa was in honor of St. Teresa of Avila and Francis was for St. Francis of Assisi.

The next name was Sabari. Sabari was the name of a woman saint in ancient India who realized God through her steadfast devotion to Him. It is told that she lived in a forest where many sages would perform great acts of penitence and complicated rituals. Sabari had a more simple form of devotion. She swept the forest pathways so that if the Lord came walking by he wouldn't get a thorn in his foot. When the local sages asked her what she was doing they laughed at her reply. But when the Lord did finally visit the forest it was to her that He came and not to those who thought of rituals instead of the Lord Himself.

The last name was the hardest one for me to get. But finally when it presented itself it felt totally right: Kaivalya.

Positive Flow Childbirth

Kaivalya is the word in Sanskrit that expresses the state of absolute oneness with God. It is a lofty goal, but one that I feel affirmed every time I say my son's name. Although, as it often happens in life, Kaivalya's name has been spontaneously shortened through affection and ease of pronunciation to Kai.

So then we had them; names that seem so natural now that we can't imagine using any others: Sabari and Kai.

No matter where your inspiration leads you in naming your child, make sure that you have given it careful consideration. It is a subtle but powerful stamp that you put on your child. And then every time you say that beautiful name, infuse it with your very best wishes for health, happiness and closeness to God.

Chapter 33

Positive Flow Childbirth

In this era of specialization it is easy to think that we can compartmentalize life and that childbirth is somehow off in a corner by itself. We are easily distracted by life's diversity and then think that everything in life is separate. I am reminded of that story I told at the very beginning about the first birth that I attended. In that moment I felt powerfully connected to life's elemental creative force in a way that I had never before experienced. The essential truth of trying to approach life in a positive spiritual way is to recognize that life's wondrous eternal magnificence is always present. It is our challenge to hold onto and deepen our awareness of this truth.

The key component to spiritualizing childbirth or in fact every part of life is to live always in the light of God's Presence even if we can't quite see it. So much of our suffering in this world comes from the feeling that we are separate from our creator. We wander from experience to experience hoping for an ultimate fulfillment, knowing instinctively that it is slipping between our fingers.

All of the great souls throughout history who have realized their oneness with God say that we are not separate from God. We have only clouded our ability to perceive that reality because

Positive Flow Childbirth

our attention is stuck in the senses. By immersing our minds in the fulfilling of desires through the senses we lose sight of the Divine Light that is always shinning upon us and through us.

So often it happens that as we seek to reclaim our divine birthright as children of God we define ourselves as weaknesses and failures. We must try constantly to remember that God's view of this world is much greater than our own human perspective. In Spirit it doesn't matter how many mistakes we make, what matters is which way we are going. Are we going towards the light of Spirit or are we moving away into the darkness of worldly consciousness. This is the only thing that really matters. For if we are going towards greater attunement to God's Will then it can only be a matter of time before we achieve our goal of conscious oneness with infinite Spirit.

So as you enter into the adventure of helping to bring a soul into this physical world remember that the light of Spirit is always shinning upon you. Endeavor to walk in that light on each step of your journey. If the darkness tries to crowd its way in then don't try to beat at it with emotions of disappointment and discouragement, defeat the darkness in life by turning on the light through the joys of spiritual activity and association.

Meditate regularly. Read spiritually uplifting books - especially about the lives of saints. Spend time with others on your spiritual path. This fellowship is of great value. And most importantly, keep company with God.

Whatever you are doing, wherever you are going, take with you the thought of God. Like a constant companion keep an inner conversation going inside your heart. Be sure to share all of your ups and downs, your questions, your deepest needs, your sorrows and joys. And don't do all of the talking! Spend time listening to the Heavenly reply, for it is there, speaking through all of life around us, and most importantly, quietly within us.

It is through divine intuition that we will ultimately experience the reality of our true nature as Spirit. This intuitive perception is the most direct communication line that we have with God. By magnetizing ourselves through our spiritual practices we begin to open up these inner lines of perception and realization. There is nothing that we can do that is more beneficial to ourselves, our children and the world in general, than the cultivation of our inner relationship with God

It is in the awareness of God's presence that we will find the solution to every challenge. If we include God in everything that we do the veil of separation will begin to dissolve and we will see more clearly than anything that we have ever seen before that we are all truly children of God.

May the Divine Light ever shine upon us. May we never turn away from that heavenly vision and may we share it with all whom we meet.

More books
by Lawrence Vijay Girard
(Nayaswami Vijay)

Way of the Positive Flow

Positive Flow Parenting

Meditation:
The Science and Art of Stillness

Flowing in the Workplace:
A Guide to Personal and
Professional Success

Stress Solutions

The Journey of Discipleship
Book 1 - Traveling with Swamiji

The Adventures of
Harry Fruitgarden
Series
Book #1 - What's it All About?
Book #2 - Who Would Have Guessed?
Book #3 - Someone Should Have Told Me!

Ask us about
Positive Flow Seminars
with Lawrence Vijay Girard

www.FruitgardenPublishing.com